Regulating Doctors

Regulating Doctors

David Gladstone (Editor)
James Johnson
William G. Pickering
Brian Salter
Meg Stacey

Institute for the Study of Civil Society
London

First published June 2000

© The Institute for the Study of Civil Society 2000
email: books@civil-society.org.uk

ISBN 1-903 386-01-2

Typeset by the Institute for the Study of Civil Society
in New Century Schoolbook

Printed in Great Britain by
St Edmundsbury Press
Bury St Edmunds, Suffolk

Contents

The Authors

David Gladstone is Director of Studies in Social Policy in the School for Policy Studies at the University of Bristol. He has published extensively on British social policy past and present. Recent titles include: *British Social Welfare, Past, Present and Future*, UCL Press, 1995; *Before Beveridge: Welfare Before the Welfare State* (ed.), IEA, 1999; *The Twentieth Century Welfare State,* Macmillan, 1999. In addition, David Gladstone is General Series Editor of Historical Sources in Social Welfare, Routledge/Thoemmes Press, and of the Open University Press' Introducing Social Policy Series. He lectures widely on aspects of British welfare history and has held several visiting professorships, especially in the USA.

James Johnson is a consultant vascular surgeon, and postgraduate clinical tutor at Halton General Hospital, Runcorn. He took office as chairman of the Joint Consultants Committee (JCC) in November 1998, having served as vice-chairman of the JCC from November 1994. The Joint Consultants Committee was set up in 1948 by the royal medical colleges and the BMA as a committee able to speak for the consultant body with one voice. The JCC represents the medical profession in discussions with the Department of Health on matters relating to the maintenance of standards of professional knowledge and skill in the hospital service and the encouragement of education and research. Members include the presidents of the medical royal colleges and their faculties and representatives from the BMA's consultants and junior doctors committees. Mr Johnson was chairman of the BMA Central Consultants and Specialists Committee from October 1994 to October 1998, and was also a previous chairman of the Junior Doctors Committee. He is also currently a member of the BMA Council.

William G. Pickering is a medical practitioner and medico-legal adviser. He qualified at Kings College Hospital in 1973 and has worked in general medicine, paediatrics and general practice. He has also had experience of medico-legal practice, having been involved in the preparation of reports for both plaintiffs and defendants in legal actions. He has a longstanding interest in the question of whether or not patients benefit from particular medical interventions, and also in the issue of ill-health caused by doctors' treatments. He has been published in many leading medical journals on these and other topics. His first published work on the need for a medical inspectorate was an article entitled 'Glasnost and the medical inspectorate' (*Journal of the Royal College of General Practitioners*, November 1988, pp. 517-18). As well as the clinical issues and the questions regarding quality control in medicine which an inspectorate raises, he is also interested in more common questions of medical ethics.

Brian Salter is Professor of Health Services Research at the University of East Anglia. He is a public policy analyst who has published widely on health and education policy matters. Recent titles include: *Oxford, Cambridge and the Changing Ideas of a University*, Open University Press, 1992; *The State and Higher Education*, Woburn Press, 1994 and *The Politics of Change in the Health Service*, Macmillan, 1998.

Meg Stacey, Emerita Professor of Sociology of the University of Warwick, has taught and researched in the sociology of health and health care for about 30 years, initially researching issues around the welfare of children in hospital. She has published widely in health matters. She has served on local and national bodies, including the (former) Hospital Management Committee in Swansea, the South Warwickshire Community Health Council and the South Warwickshire Maternity Services Liaison Committee, and the (former) Welsh Hospital Board, as well as the General Medical Council. She sat on the latter from 1976-1983 and subsequently researched it with support from the Economic and Social Research Council and the Leverhulme Trust. Alert to moral and social issues in medical practice, she is currently active in the independent Human Values in Health Care Forum.

Foreword

The conviction of the GP, Harold Shipman, for murdering several of his patients was taken as evidence that something was fundamentally wrong with medical regulation, and both the Government and the General Medical Council (GMC) have conceded that reform is necessary. However, the real problem is self-regulation itself, which allows the organised medical profession to exploit monopoly power. Indeed, for nearly a hundred years the GMC has functioned, not only as the guardian of medical ethics, but also as the enforcer of a trade-union rule book. The root of the problem lies in changes made at the beginning of the twentieth century.

Towards the end of the nineteenth century doctors were keen to distinguish their profession from 'trade'. A profession, doctors claimed, enforced higher standards than the minimalist 'honesty is the best policy' pragmatism of the market. But did it? In truth there have been two traditions within the medical profession. One saw medicine as a vocation, and insisted on a code of ethics which prohibited doctors from putting their interests above those of their patients. The other regarded medicine as a 'guild' passing on the 'mystery' of medicine from generation to generation and showing solidarity against outsiders. The GMC continues to reflect both these traditions.

The origins of the General Medical Council lie in the Medical Act of 1858 which empowered it to erase a doctor from the medical register if he was found guilty of 'infamous conduct in any professional respect'. Some doctors took the view that it constituted 'infamous conduct' to fail to co-operate with professional restrictive practices intended to limit competition and raise fees.

Several members of the GMC argued that it would be *ultra vires* for it to protect the 'pecuniary interests' of doctors. However, the GMC came under strong pressure from medical militants and a resolution passed in July 1899 by the County of Durham Medical Union reveals their 'guild' mentality:

> That when the Qualified Practitioners of any district make a combined effort to raise the standard of their fees, and thereby the status of the profession, it should be deemed infamous conduct in a professional respect for any Registered Practitioner to attempt to frustrate their efforts by opposing them at cheaper rates of payment, and canvassing for patients.

In 1902 the GMC succumbed to these pressures and outlawed advertising, the chief means of attracting new patients. The case in question concerned a doctor who had issued handbills in a poor district of Birmingham. Initially he had announced that he would provide a free service for the poor, but he was so inundated by the response that he found it necessary to issue a second circular advertising a small charge of 3d, much lower than the going rate. The Medical Defence Union led the case against him and told the GMC that the circulars had been issued with one intention only: to take patients from other 'medical men'. The GMC had resisted such pressures for many years, but in 1902 it caved in and banned advertising.

That the GMC was being openly used to further the pecuniary interests of doctors at the expense of patients was well understood at the time. There was much press interest, including accusations that the GMC had become an instrument of 'trade-unionism'. Competition was no longer something which might lead to social ostracism by the medial fraternity, it could now cost you your job, and the BMA was not slow to point this out to 'blacklegs'.

The philosophy behind the GMC is to protect consumers by issuing a licence only to doctors who have undergone a standardised programme of education. Before the GMC was founded in 1858 there were 21 licensing bodies, and to some commentators this seemed like chaos. However, we can now see more clearly that there was merit in competition between organisations upholding different standards. The reality of a single standard has not been that bad doctors have been eliminated, but quite the opposite. Bad doctors, and in extreme cases even criminals, have been shielded from normal accountability. Without the official seal of approval of the GMC, doctors would have to rely on their reputation, technical competence, character and personal qualities to attract patients. But so long as they are on the medical register, and so long as the medical register is controlled by fellow doctors who can be counted on to be lenient in virtually all circumstances, they are safe from serious scrutiny.

As in so many spheres, concentrated monopoly power is the underlying problem, and the safest remedy would be to abolish the GMC. Without the GMC we could expect a variety of agencies to emerge giving their own seal of approval to doctors and hospitals. The royal colleges would undoubtedly play a part, perhaps consumer organisations might get involved, or maybe health insurers would provide a seal of approval, just as car insurers maintain an approved list of vehicle repairers. Such diversity would be more likely to foster the tradition of medicine as a vocation which has been diminished, but by no means destroyed, by the corrosive influence of officially-sanctioned monopoly.

Each in their own way, the contributors to this book struggle with the same problem and each offers a different solution. But while there is, as yet, no agreement about the best strategy for reform, there is now a wide consensus that the regulation of the medical profession cannot be left as it is.

But far more is at stake than is implied by the contest between champions of self-regulation and advocates of consumer control. A free society depends for its vitality on the existence of organisations which are independent of the political process, so that when political parties submit their manifestos for appraisal by public opinion, there is a truly independent body of opinion capable of standing in judgement, and not merely a mass of individuals who have been manipulated by the technicians of 'news management'. Historically the professions have been prominent among the organisations which have provided the strong voices capable of serving as bulwarks against the undue concentration of political power. The authority of the medical profession rested partly on science but also on public respect for the tradition of medicine as a vocation. Today, the challenge is to discover how best to rebuild this spirit. The issue touches not only upon the machinery of regulation, but also the extent to which clinical judgement has been eroded as doctors have become more like Treasury gatekeepers and less the champions of the patient. An independent profession, inspired by service, and determined to put patients first, should not be content to submit to central direction. For far too long many NHS doctors have been willing to remain silent while they withheld or delayed clinically necessary treatments on financial grounds. GPs, in particular, have become progressively more like salaried government employees than independent professionals and, although it will strike many as counter-intuitive, abolishing the GMC is among the measures necessary to reinvigorate the tradition of medicine as a vocation.

David G. Green

Editor's Introduction

Regulation, Accountability and Health Care

David Gladstone

In the last two decades the position of the medical profession appears to have changed. The corporate power of medicine has been increasingly challenged and doctors, the high priests of modern society, have become increasingly embattled as their position as experts has been challenged from inside and outside the health care arena.[1]

Medical self-regulation is under scrutiny and very firmly back on the political and professional agenda. That renewed attention and re-examination owes much to the conviction of Dr Harold Shipman, and to the 'Bristol case' to which Stacey, Salter and Pickering refer in their essays in this collection. That case is currently the subject of a public inquiry appointed in late 1998 by the Secretary of State for Health and chaired by Professor Ian Kennedy. Its on-going deliberations have generated considerable publicity. So too did the hearings conducted by the General Medical Council (GMC) against the medical personnel involved. The cumulative impact has been to raise concern about medical self-regulation, and the related issues of accountability and quality in health care.

That concern was dramatically focused at the end of January 2000 by the conviction, after a lengthy trial, of Dr Harold Shipman, a general practitioner in Greater Manchester, who had been accused of the murder of 15 of his female patients. In his statement to the House of Commons on the day following Dr Shipman's conviction, the Secretary of State for Health announced the appointment of an independent inquiry. Part of the remit of that inquiry concerns the processes of the General Medical Council—the medical profession's self-regulatory body—and the political aspiration that it will more transparently work in the interests of patients rather than doctors. In the Secretary of State's words:

The GMC ... must be truly accountable and it must be guided at all times by the welfare and safety of patients. We owe it to the relatives of Shipman's victims to prevent a repetition of what happened in Hyde.[2]

1

The Bristol case and the Shipman conviction have given undoubted public prominence to the issues of quality and accountability in health care, just as they have highlighted the need to restore confidence in the doctor/patient relationship. But, as the quotation at the head of this Introduction suggestively argues, the challenge to medical professional power and self-regulation has a significant pre-history. Over the past two decades it has been the subject of considerable attention both from within the medical profession itself and as the result of a whole variety of external factors.

The broader context is, of course, 'the backlash against professional society'. As Perkin defines it, this reaction operated at three levels:

• against the power, privileges and pretensions of special interest groups ... especially the organised professions;

• against the seemingly unstoppable growth of 'big government' with the attempt to 'roll back the state' by cutting public expenditure and privatising nationalised industries;

• against corporatism, the involvement of special interest groups, above all employers and trade unions, in the framing of government policy.[3]

It is hardly surprising that the medical profession became part of this backlash against professional society, given their social status, specialist knowledge and predominant—though not exclusive —employment in the public sector. The challenges were many and various: the internal market with its separation of purchasing and provider functions; citizens' charters, quality assurance and the introduction of greater managerial responsibility into professional practice with increased surveillance of activity, assessment of spending and measures of outcome expressed in indicators such as league tables, medical audit and indicative drugs budgets. Improving the quality of health care, enhancing consumer choice and providing value for money were the keynotes of successive Conservative governments in the 1980s and 1990s. In practice, it appeared that medical auton-omy was under threat, and that a new concordat was being forged between the state and the medical profession.[4] Studies of policy change frequently highlight that what is left off the agenda is as impor-tant—and sometimes more so—than what is included. That observation is particularly pertinent in the case of the introduction of the internal market reforms in 1990. At that time, as Salter notes, 'the state made no attempt to challenge the basis of medical power: the principle of self-regulation itself' (p. 14).

Quality is also an integral feature of New Labour's programme for the NHS, and the measures it has taken to promote it betoken further change for the medical profession in its relationship with the state.

These measures include:

- the inauguration of the National Institute for Clinical Excellence (NICE) designed to give authoritative advice to health professionals on the best treatment for their patients;

- the introduction of National Service Frameworks to set national standards, and the imposition on local health services of a legal duty of quality;

- the inception of a new Commission for Health Improvement charged with the responsibility for monitoring the performance of every part of the NHS.

For New Labour these initiatives represent important ingredients in the creation of a modern and dependable NHS. But, as Salter notes, there are other implications:

> Once the state is publicly acknowledged to have responsibility for at least part of medicine's control of knowledge, the authority for the creation, disposal and application of that knowledge no longer resides solely with the profession. Further, if the authority on which the legitimacy of clinical decisions rests is no longer wholly internal to the profession, but ultimately is derived from the new clinical governance responsibilities of the state, from what source does covert clinical rationing ... then derive *its* justification? (p. 16).

Together, therefore, Shipman's conviction, the Bristol case and the changes just reviewed—not to mention a more articulate consumerism in health care—represent a significant challenge to the idea and practice of medical self-regulation. It is this context of quality and accountability which gives a topicality and importance to the essays in this collection.

The changing contours of medical self-regulation form the basis of the essays by Salter and Stacey. Both of them allude to the origins of the practice, established by the Medical Act of 1858, whereby 'the state ratified medicine's claims to be an autonomous self-governing ethical profession'.[5] In return there was the guarantee that the service provided would be of a satisfactory standard. This was to be achieved in two ways. First, by confirming the status of approved practitioners as recorded in the register of the General Medical Council to those who had been appropriately educated, trained and licensed to practise. Secondly, by the decision of the professional conduct committee of the GMC to remove a doctor from the register for what was deemed to be 'serious professional misconduct'. Essentially this was a reactive process. Since 1995, however, through the performance review procedures, the GMC has introduced new systems which are more pro-active. The performance review procedures are designed to enhance the Council's ability both to detect and correct inappropriate standards in clinical care.

They also suggest a range of corrective actions to be taken once the nature of a doctor's poor performance has been established. Both the essays by Salter and Johnson allude to the role of continuing medical professional education and re-training in this process; though Salter indicates that there is still a long way to go before a system is achieved that is 'consistent, comprehensive and mandatory, and seen to be so' (p. 22).

Stacey provides an excellent incisive narrative of recent developments within the GMC (of which she was for a period a lay member) and discusses—as does Salter—initiatives from within the profession that are designed to show that medical self-regulation can work to restore public confidence and trust. Drawing on her own research, published earlier in the 1990s, she comments that '[t]he GMC had always been slow to examine the clinical aspects of complaints and reluctant to accept that serious incompetence amounted to SPM (serious professional misconduct)' (p. 34). That situation, she believes, has changed. Over recent years, in her view, both the GMC and the medical profession have become more pro-active in their approach to medical self-regulation. It is possible to argue that such change is the product of a variety of factors. On the one hand, it represents a means for the medical profession to regain public confidence. On the other, it can be seen as an attempt to forestall a greater degree of external (i.e. governmental) control and surveillance over professional activity. Alternatively, of course, the introduction of new procedures within the profession can be seen as a route to both objectives. Paradoxically, therefore, as Stacey observes, the short-term consequences have not been particularly salutary, satisfying neither profession nor public. Public suspicion of the GMC and of the medical profession in general appears to have increased as a result of the Bristol case, while more doctors than ever before see the GMC as punitive (p. 36).

The essays by Johnson and Pickering concentrate on the means by which the medical profession might become more accountable. From his perspective within the medical profession, Johnson's context is of a profession which he believes to be baffled and wounded by the attacks made upon it. It is against that background that he argues the need for a more explicit partnership to be established between the GMC and the profession in order to 'roll out effective self-regulation into the workplace' (p. 41). As part of that process, his essay highlights four inter-related components of a more pro-active programme of self-regulation. These are the greater use of outcome data, peer review and appraisal, revalidation (i.e. retraining) and continuing professional education and development. There is much here that suggests an enhanced role for peer professional appraisal. But his essay also contains a message for the GMC as an institution in the triangle of political forces in health care that Salter identified. In investigating the under-performance of individual practitioners it must be equally willing 'to point the finger at inadequate funding, poor facilities and excessive workload' (p. 46). Quality standards, that is to say, are not only about competence but the conditions that enable or restrict the abilities of the individual practitioner. That is a message for government which many professionals in other sectors will readily endorse.

Pickering's essay appears to go beyond the pattern of established organisations, with his call for the setting up of a medical inspectorate to provide informed and independent assessment of what he terms 'sub-standard clinical practice' (p. 47).

Inspectorates have a considerable history in British social policy programmes—the Education and Factory Inspectorate for example, as well as the more recent Social Services Inspectorate—often being associated with the Benthamite-inspired 'nineteenth century revolution in government'. Pickering does not specifically set out the administrative arrangements he has in mind for his proposed inspectorate, but his discussion of the dental reference officers provides what is quite clearly an important analogy. In his terms, they serve as a quality inspectorate carrying out quality monitoring of dental services. The introduction of such a scheme into medical practice, Pickering believes, would raise clinical standards, improve staff morale and enhance patient confidence in medical competence.

Though sceptical of its usefulness as a measure of equality, it is Pickering alone of the contributors to this collection who specifically discusses patient satisfaction (pp. 58-59). Such a focus serves to remind us that quality and accountability are multi-faceted and that patient (or user) evaluation may be based on a variety of often undifferentiated factors. Stewart's discussion, for example, indicated the different forms of accountability:

- management accountability—the accountability of managers to their supervisors in the organisation;

- professional accountability—the accountability of professionals to the standards of their profession as enforced by professional associations;

- contractual accountability which is playing an increasing role in the welfare system and refers to accountability in terms of the contract;

- client or user accountability—the direct account—to the individuals who receive the service.[6]

In Stewart's terms, much of the discussion in this collection centres upon professional accountability and its interface with other (especially managerial) elements in the triangle of political forces in health care. There is a danger, however, that such a perspective may minimise the dynamics of the doctor/patient interaction and the issues of quality and accountability that arise between them in that context. Studies of patienthood in practice have suggested that each may bring uncertainty to the encounter: the uncertainty of symptoms and the treatment regime on the one hand; the uncertainty of medical knowledge on the other. If the former leads, at least for Pickering, to unreasonable demands on the medical profession (p. 59), the latter may lead doctors to use information control in what is disclosed to patients. It underlines the point made by Johnson which bears significantly on the issue of accountability, that 'at the end of the twentieth century diagnosis is often no more than an educated guess based on physical findings and medical tests, the results of which are frequently contradictory' (pp. 40-41). But it is also well-established that each of the partners in the doctor/patient encounter may have different expectations.

> To the patient the reason for the consultation may be pressing and intimate and personally crucial (while) to the doctor it represents no more than a brief exchange, a drop in an ocean of symptoms to be dealt with as part of routine work.[7]

It is, of course, formal complaints which provide at least some evidence of levels of patient satisfaction or dissatisfaction. But what is the patient and consumer view of what constitutes effectiveness and satisfaction? To put it another way, what do patients complain about? The mechanisms for complaints are diverse and the literature on the topic is limited, but in a study of 110 complaints about general practitioners adjudicated by a health authority, Allsop suggested that they overwhelmingly combined allegations of technical failure and allegations relating to codes of behaviour. 'Technical failures' encompassed access to the doctor, an inadequate examination, a wrong diagnosis, inappropriate treatment (including drug prescribing) and a lack of referral to another health worker. Allegations relating to behaviour included describing the doctor as disinterested or rude, cruel or threatening. In the context of Dr Pickering's focus on substandard clinical practice as the remit of his medical inspectorate, it is interesting, as Allsop's account makes clear, that, for the patient, technical failures and the nature of the consultation cannot be so readily distinguished.[8] In her investigation, the one was usually accompanied by the other.

This introduction has deliberately sought to locate the discussion of medical self-regulation within the context of the broader debate about quality and accountability in health care. In that context it is interesting to note that over the past six years complaints against doctors have risen three-fold and that currently the GMC has a backlog of 160 disciplinary cases awaiting decision. That raises issues about the procedures of medicine's self-regulating body. But, as the Secretary of State indicated in his speech establishing the independent inquiry, the issue is also one of re-establishing the relationship of trust between patient and their medical practitioner both in primary care and in the hospital sector.

It is pertinent to inquire how far the GMC's own proposals for change, agreed at its meeting in early February 2000, will achieve that objective. Thus far they have received a cautious welcome. Those proposals include greater lay representation including on its fitness-to-practise committees and the power to suspend immediately doctors who are suspected of criminal offences or incompetence. Such changes have been under discussion for four years. It is difficult not to conclude that the GMC has reached a decision at this juncture only under the considerable adverse publicity occasioned by the Shipman trial and the Bristol inquiry and out of a concern that political pressure may yet impose a more rigorous regulatory regime.

Implicit—and to some degree explicit—in all of this is whether doctors alone are competent to judge the decisions of fellow medics against whom complaints may be brought. But the issue also concerns whether a body whose legal responsibilities were established in the very different world of nineteenth century medicine has any continuing relevance in the vastly changed conditions of contemporary health care. Part of the onus on those inquiring into the wider implications of recent tragic cases must be to identify what—if any—that continuing role may be and how an organisation that has been so closely identified with the protection of its members can become more transparently effective in working for patients.

Change in the Governance of Medicine: The Politics of Self-Regulation

Brian Salter

Introduction

Since the creation of the General Medical Council (GMC) by the 1858 Medical Act, medicine's system of governance has been based on the principle of state-sanctioned self-regulation. Historically, that principle was not questioned by the state but accepted as the necessary lynchpin of a socio-political bargain that it was in the common interest of medicine, civil society and the state to uphold. However, under the pressure of recent events, coupled with wider shifts in the political culture, civil society and the state have become more sceptical of the benefits of self-regulation and more insistent that change in the governance of medicine should take place.

To an extent, the medical profession has recognised and responded to the need for change, though it is doubtful whether the reforms it has introduced thus far are sufficient to ensure the continuation of its professional autonomy in its traditional form. The mounting demands for accountability and openness are too great, and further change is inevitable. However, it is far from clear how such change can be introduced, or what impact any reformulation of the principle of self-regulation would have on the state or indeed on society itself. What is apparent is that the tensions in the triangular relationship between medicine, civil society and the state are too complex to be susceptible to the instructions of simple policy *fiat*.

The objective of this chapter is to identify the nature of those tensions and their impact on the politics of self-regulation, using a three-stage approach. First, an analytical framework is developed which provides an understanding of how the political forces of the triangular relationship interact to guide and constrain change in medicine's system of governance. Building on that understanding, the pressures for change on the different spheres of medical self-regulation are examined and their interdependence explored. Third, the existing and likely response of medicine's self-regulating bodies is analysed to determine how far their traditional, and largely informal, approach to

8

the politics of change will be sufficient to deal with the array of political demands they now face. Fourth, change is not without its costs, and the final section explores the political price the profession may have to pay if self-regulation is to remain a reality.

Self-regulation And The Triangle Of Forces

The governance of medicine, that is the ways in which the profession is held accountable for its actions, is by no means synonymous with self-regulation. External regulation of the profession occurs through NHS procedures, the legal framework (e.g. on medical negligence), and watchdogs such as the Mental Health Commission and the Health Service Commissioner.[1] However, none of these mechanisms intrude on the core identity of the profession, derived as this is from its control of medical knowledge. The right to govern the definition, disposal and application of medical knowledge without recourse to an external authority has, since the foundation of the GMC, been construed as a purely internal professional matter and has constituted the rock on which medical power has been built. It follows, as Stacey has observed, that:

> there is a rather special form of public accountability inherent in professional self-regulation; individual professionals are accountable to their individual patients, but a professional body is responsible for seeing that the collectivity of individual practitioners performs appropriately.[2]

As a political resource, the statutory right to self-regulation has proved invaluable and has enabled the profession to negotiate numerous advantageous arrangements with its economic and political environment regarding, for example, the regulation of its members' market entry and exit, competitive practices and remuneration.[3]

In return for the statutory right to self-regulate its own knowledge territory, medicine acknowledged its duty to ensure that, in terms of both education and practice, its use of that knowledge would be in the public interest.[4] In the words of the Merrison Report on the regulation of the medical profession, self-regulation is:

> a contract between the public and the profession, by which the public go to the profession for medical treatment because the profession has made sure it will provide satisfactory treatment.[5]

Provided the profession retains the trust of the public, then it also fulfils the terms of its contract with the state and self-regulation can continue unhindered. But if the profession fails in its task, then parliament must act to protect the citizens on whose behalf it originally ceded the privilege of self-regulation when it established the GMC. Not to do so would constitute a failure by the state to fulfil the terms of its own contract with civil society—that is, the delivery of the healthcare rights enshrined in British citizenship.

The three contracts between medicine, civil society and the state interlock to form a triangle of forces based on a mutual exchange of political benefits (figure 1).

Figure 1: The Triangle of Political Forces

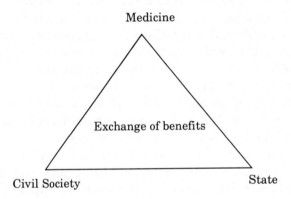

The political benefits are:

For civil society
- citizenship healthcare rights from the state
- delivered by health care of an appropriate standard by medicine

For the state
- rationing of healthcare resources by medicine
- respect for the state's authority and legitimacy from society

For medicine
- trust from society
- the privilege of self-regulation from the state

The interdependence of the contracts and the political benefits they produce ensures that difficulties with one contract inevitably create problems for the other two. This in turn means that the political management of change in different areas of the triangle of forces has to be orchestrated and the repercussions of individual policy actions anticipated. If this is not done, then the stability of the triangle of forces as a whole is threatened and all parties to the arrangement risk losing their present benefits.

The viability of the three-way bargain is dependent upon the network of institutions which operate medicine's system of self-regulation.[6]

Their task is to guarantee that the profession's control of medical knowledge is conducted according to standards acceptable to civil society and the state. Within this network, although the GMC has statutory responsibility for both education and performance monitoring, it is reliant upon numerous other centres of medical power for the delivery of both functions (e.g. medical royal colleges, university medical schools, British Medical Association).[7] Given that these different medical organisations make overlapping contributions to the process of self-regulation, political tensions between them are not uncommon, particularly when they are subject to pressures for change.[8] Nonetheless, through the use of informal ties of custom and practice, élite co-ordinating bodies such as the Joint Consultants Committee (JCC) and brokerage institutions such as the Academy of Medical Royal Colleges, change in the system of self-regulation has been achieved, albeit slowly. What remains to be seen is how far this traditional approach to the management of change can cope with the rapidly rising tide of demand for improvements in medicine's internal governance.

The Pressures For Change

The pressures for change are analysed in terms of the three dimensions of the triangle of forces, the political benefits at risk within each, and the consequent implications for the mechanisms of self-regulation.

Medicine and civil society

Society's questioning of the principle and practice of medicine's unique control of medical knowledge is a well established phenomenon. The proponents of the 'de-professionalisation thesis' have argued for some time that there has been a general decline in the profession's cultural authority and legitimacy,[9] that the rise of complementary medicine is a clear indication of the erosion of that authority,[10] that technology has increased the accessibility of medical knowledge to non-doctors, that medicine has become reliant upon new areas of knowledge which it does not control,[11] and that the preparedness of patients to challenge doctors' decisions is reflected in the steady rise in complaints about medical care and the prominence of patient lobby groups on the national political stage.[12] However the translation of these cultural shifts into specific political pressure on self-regulation has until recently lacked a suitable vehicle.

The high profile case of the three Bristol consultants disciplined by the GMC for professional misconduct and the associated public inquiry has supplied such a vehicle and created a political issue with substantial and probably enduring impetus.[13] As Klein points out:

Bristol represents a landmark in the history of self-regulation of the medical profession in the UK in terms of its length, its salience in the eyes of the public, and the issues it has raised.[14]

By providing an emotive focal point for the expression of public doubt about the competence of doctors, the Bristol case has politicised self-regulation. Three years ago Sir Donald Irvine, then newly appointed as President of the GMC, commented with some prescience:

> Self-regulation in any system—be it medicine or parliament—is built on trust. And if a gap grows between those who are regulating themselves and the public they serve—that's when the threat to self-regulation comes.[15]

That gap is now publicly acknowledged and the threat to medicine's twin political benefits of public trust and self-regulation is starkly apparent. Klein may be correct in his observation concerning the Bristol case that:

> If there were any doubts about the GMC's commitment to its contract with the public, about its determination to demonstrate the profession's collective acceptance of responsibility for maintaining competence in practice, they have been dispelled.[16]

Unfortunately, the problem lies not with the GMC's commitment but with the inability of the existing mechanisms of self-regulation to reassure the public.

Civil society and the state

If medicine has a problem, so does the state. The right to free health care from the cradle to the grave is an integral part of British citizenship which it is the duty of the state to fulfil. As the concept of what constitutes health and the range of possible treatments have expanded, so the legitimate demands of citizens on the NHS have increased. So much so that, from the very foundation of the NHS, demand has always outstripped supply.[17] The relationship between demand and supply in any area of activity is normally controlled by the application of a cost to the expression of the demand but, given that this was ideologically unacceptable to the NHS, an alternative mechanism had to be found. Since 'implicit in the structure of the NHS' was a bargain between medicine and the state which ensured that 'while central government controlled the budget, doctors controlled what happened within that budget',[18] it was inevitable that, in their disposal of NHS resources, doctors would have to perform the necessary rationing function of balancing the demand/supply equation if the system was not to collapse. This function has always been covert in the sense that it is embedded within the normal course of clinical decision-making.

Medicine's ability to carry out this key political task is dependent upon the public's trust in the competence of clinicians. Once that trust is undermined, so is medicine's efficacy as a rationing agent. If clinical autonomy and the system of self-regulation which maintains it are seen, not as a guarantee of impartial and competent medical treatment regardless of cost, but as an ideological cloak for professional protectionism, then the state has lost the principal political instrument for convincing its citizens that their rights are being delivered. Once that happens, either the state has to find another mechanism, acceptable to its citizens, for dealing with the perennial demand/supply mismatch, or it will find that societal respect for its authority will diminish.[19]

The difficulty with all explicit rationing mechanisms is that they are a public denial of someone's, or some group's, healthcare rights—a situation unacceptable to the NHS principle of universality.[20] By definition, therefore, such mechanisms can be immediately challenged with the result that:

> explicit rationing is inevitably unstable because of the ability of small groups to evoke public sympathy and support in contesting government decision-making ... [thus] pushing the health system towards more flexible implicit approaches.[21]

Unless, or until, the state is prepared to redefine its citizens' healthcare rights and the associated NHS ideology, or to expand the supply of healthcare resources on an unprecedented and unknowable scale, it must remain dependent upon covert rationing by the medical profession as the means for managing its relationship with civil society.

Medicine and the state

The state's dependence on medicine for the resolution of the demand/supply conundrum in health care found its original expression in the corporatist agreement between medicine and the state which accompanied the creation of universal healthcare rights with the foundation of the NHS in 1948.[22] That agreement gave the profession power over the disposal of NHS resources, the ability 'to veto policy change by defining the limits of the acceptable and by determining the policy agenda',[23] and confirmation of medicine's right to self-regulation.[24] Over the succeeding decades the arrangement consolidated into a form of 'ideological corporatism' which ensured that policy was framed within a set of values acceptable to this particular knowledge élite to produce what some have regarded as an example of 'the professionalised state'.[25] Confirmation, if confirmation were needed, of medicine's uniquely powerful position within the Health Service came with the publication of the Merrison Report on the regulation of the medical profession, which reasserted the advantages to society of a self-determining knowledge élite.[26]

Yet, with the arrival of the 1980s, the apparent inevitability of the state's subordination to medicine was abruptly challenged. Successive Conservative governments, heavily influenced by the thinking of the New Right,[27] developed a view of healthcare provision which emphasised the importance of consumer choice, the elimination of professional barriers to the operation of the market, and positive public management in the delivery of health care. To such an ideology, the medical profession's 'self-regulation based on trust among gentlemen was an inadequate guiding principle for public policy',[28] the corporatist 'politics of the double bed' an anachronism,[29] and the need for a realignment of the relationship between medicine, civil society and the state self-evident.

Much to the medical profession's chagrin, the overhaul of the medicine/state relationship duly took place with the promotion of NHS managers as a power group to rival the doctors, the erosion of the established 'iron triangle' of the medical profession, officials and ministers,[30] the abolition of medicine's policy veto and its exclusion from the inner sanctum of policy making from the 1988 Review of the NHS onwards, and, as the doctors' wounded surprise turned to anger, a series of acrimonious disputes between the profession's leaders and successive secretaries of state for health.[31]

Yet, although significant aspects of the original corporatist agreement were dismantled, the state made no attempt to challenge the basis of medical power: the principle of self-regulation itself. *Working for Patients*, the white paper which initiated the 1991 reforms, emphasised that 'the quality of medical work should be reviewed by a doctor's peers',[32] and medicine's autonomous system of professional governance continued on its serene course, largely unhindered by the storms afflicting the NHS's formal accountability structures. Indeed, by the mid-1990s it looked as though the state had learnt the error of its ways, realised its fundamental dependence upon the medical profession's demand-control function, publicly transformed the managers from heroes to villains, and was returning to a grudging acceptance of the medical hegemony.[33]

However, the state's acceptance was tinged with an awareness that self-regulation might itself require reform. Muted though it may have been, from the late 1980s onwards there had been pressure from the Privy Council and ministers for the GMC to rethink its professional misconduct procedures.[34] This pressure was focused in 1993 when problems with South Birmingham's pathology service caused the Secretary of State for Health to request a review by the department's chief medical officer (CMO) of guidance in relation to the identification of poor performance of doctors.[35] Given that the majority of the Review Group were leading members of medicine's élites, its subsequent report *Maintaining Medical Excellence* can be viewed as a clear recognition by the profession that the pressures from the state were real and required a tangible response.

At this time, the state's attitude did not evoke any sense of great urgency: change was necessary but did not demand drastic measures. However, with the arrival of the 1997 Labour government, the state has taken a new and, from medicine's perspective, challenging direction in its approach to self-regulation. The white paper *The New NHS: Modern, Dependable* indicated that the government will seek 'to strengthen the existing systems of professional self-regulation by ensuring that they are open, responsive and publicly accountable'.[36] This was followed, first, by the announcement that 'for the first time in the history of the NHS' hospital trusts are to be held legally accountable for the quality of the service they provide;[37] and, second, by the consultation document *A First Class Service: Quality in the New NHS*, which proposes a comprehensive, management-led system of clinical governance designed to set and monitor clinical standards.[38] Self-regulation remains but the document notes that, if the public confidence dented by events such as those surrounding the Bristol consultants is to be restored, self-regulation must be modernised to ensure that it is:

> open to public scrutiny; responsive to changing clinical practice and changing service needs; and publicly accountable for professional standards set nationally and the action taken to maintain those standards.[39]

'Government', says the document, 'will take responsibility for clarifying which treatments work best'.[40]

By proposing to take ultimate responsibility for clinical standards, a key area in the control of medical knowledge, the state has announced its intention to redefine the contract between medicine and the state. It has forcefully reminded the medical profession that, in the words of the Merrison report:

> The legislature—that is, Parliament—acts in this context for the public, and it is for Parliament to decide the nature of the contract [between medicine and the public] and the way it is executed.[41]

In taking this action the state is moving to ensure that its citizens' healthcare rights are protected and hence that the terms of its citizenship contract with civil society are fulfilled.

All well and good. But what the state appears not to have considered is the likely effect of a redefinition of the terms of self-regulation, since this is what is proposed, on the stability of the triangle of political forces. Once the state is publicly acknowledged to have responsibility for at least part of medicine's control of knowledge, the authority for the creation, disposal and application of that knowledge no longer resides solely with the profession. Further, if the authority on which the legitimacy of clinical decisions rests is no longer wholly internal to the profession, but ultimately is derived from the new clinical governance responsibilities of the state, from what source does covert clinical rationing (one of the state's major political benefits from the triangular relationship) then derive *its* justification? Is the state not in danger of shooting itself in the foot by undermining the medical profession's ability to deal with the demand/supply mismatch and making itself the target for patient dissatisfaction with clinical decisions?

Managing Change

To a considerable extent, the way in which these issues develop and impact on the triangular relationship between medicine, civil society and the state will depend on the profession's ability to translate the pressures from society and state into convincing reforms of its internal governance. Its experience in this field is not vast. The profession's steady acquisition of power since the 1858 Medical Act, the concessions to medical hegemony which accompanied the foundation of the NHS, and the interlocking strength of the triangle of forces have rendered it less than appreciative of the need for change. This reluctance has been compounded by characteristics inherent in the present system of self-regulation which make change more difficult to manage effectively.

In order to understand the politics of change in that system, driven as it is by the imperatives of knowledge control, it is helpful to juxtapose: (a) the arena of knowledge control with, (b) the regulation functions necessary to achieve knowledge control (Figure 2).

Figure 2:
Knowledge Control and the Politics of Self-regulation

	Regulation Activity		
Arena of Knowledge Control	Standard setting	Monitoring and evaluation	Intervention
Creation (Research)			
Transmission (Education)			
Application (Performance			

Each cell within the matrix represents a regulatory territory over which political conflict can occur. Historically, medicine has demonstrated an ingenious capacity to evolve institutions which compete for dominance of these territories. Clearly, in order to exercise effective power over one of the three knowledge-control arenas, a particular institution, or groups of institutions, would need to combine the regulation activities of standard setting, evaluation against those standards, and intervention, into a single line of accountability or governance. In practice, this has not proved easy. Given their historic rivalries and overlapping regulation functions, institutions have found it difficult to agree not only on the nature of the proposed changes but also on the means by which they will be achieved. Change has therefore been a lengthy and incremental process. However, with the state now indicating its willingness to compete for a share in the control of the regulatory territories, the minds of the medical élites are rapidly being focused on how the profession can best manage change in the internal governance of its research, education and performance. What are their chances of success and what are the major constraints they must overcome?

Research

In order for the legitimacy of medical decisions to be sustained over time, the knowledge base for those decisions has to be seen as both valid and reliable. Traditionally the production of new medical knowledge has been governed by the tenets of scientific research and peer review which, it was assumed, were sufficient to guarantee the quality of the knowledge product. Major funding agencies such as the Medical Research Council (MRC) have their own self-regulating procedures.[42] However, of late the awareness has grown that national measures are required to define and regulate research standards in order to maintain public confidence in the findings of medical research.[43] In part, this awareness was stimulated by recent examples of misconduct in research, but in part also by the pressures so forcefully produced by the public and state response to the case of the Bristol consultants.[44] If the profession is to sustain its present impetus towards the closer integration of research and practice as enshrined in evidence-based medicine, then clearly the process of knowledge creation itself has to be seen to be beyond reproach.

As the apparatus of medical self-regulation considers the way forward in this relatively new arena of knowledge control, it would do well to reflect on the state's probable interest in it as the quality agenda of the NHS is moved forward. The proposed National Institute for Clinical Excellence (NICE), with its clinical evidence collection and appraisal functions and its incorporation of various related state-funded initiatives,[45] is likely to develop its own view of how the quality of new medical knowledge should be defined, evaluated and, where necessary, corrected.

Education

Statutory responsibility for the regulation of all stages of medical education rests with the Education Committee of the GMC. However, its ability to co-ordinate the profession's response to the pressures for change in this arena is heavily circumscribed by its need to negotiate with numerous other centres of power involved in the delivery and accreditation of education: notably, in undergraduate education, the university medical schools and the Council of Deans of UK Medical Schools and Faculties; and in postgraduate education, the medical royal colleges and faculties, the postgraduate deans, and the BMA.[46] Not only do these institutions regard the GMC's lead role with ill-disguised scepticism, they also directly control much of the standard setting, evaluation and intervention components of the medical education regulation structure. As a result, governance in this arena is fragmented and exercised through a series of institutional links, some stronger than others, which lead eventually to the GMC.

Looking now in detail at one important example of change, that of postgraduate education, the major reason why the reforms originally proposed by the Royal Commission on Medical Education in1968 (the Todd Report), and vigorously supported by the 1979 Merrison Report on the NHS, could not be implemented was because no satisfactory way was found to protect the interests of the accrediting bodies, the medical royal colleges, and they duly vetoed the reforms.[47] Subsequently, following legal pressure from the European Union, the Calman Report recommended radical changes in postgraduate training which are presently being implemented.[48] Significantly, the implementation follows agreement between the principal institutions in this arena, the royal colleges and the GMC, concerning the protection of their respective power interests. The basic components of the new agreement are that a new qualification called the Certificate of Completion of Specialist Training (CCST) is awarded by the Specialist Training Authority (STA—a joint colleges/GMC body) on the recommendation of the appropriate royal college and the name of the successful individual is then placed on the Specialist Register which is maintained and published by the GMC. Honour is thus satisfied, as is the need to maintain an appropriate balance of power between the regulating institutions.

Achieving that balance has required considerable effort behind the scenes for many years. Although the Education Committee of the GMC had by the late 1980s developed a view of the changes needed in postgraduate education,[49] it was also aware that before any action could be considered 'a pattern of working relations' with the royal colleges would have to be established as a result of 'the requirement imposed by regulation by professional consensus'.[50] Given such an approach to the management of change, it is inevitable, as Stacey observes, that 'the felt need to consult and consult again in order to reach consensus decisions greatly slows down the decision-making process'.[51]

Performance

Whether this leisurely approach will be sufficient to deal with the pressures presently experienced by self-regulation in the arena of performance (the application of medical knowledge) is a key question in the political equation, particularly given the range of institutions and their various regulatory contributions. Ultimate statutory control of professional standards is exercised through the GMC's maintenance of the register of doctors fit to practise medicine and the power of its Professional Conduct Committee to remove a doctor from that register for 'serious professional misconduct'.[52] In addition, in 1997, in the wake of the Medical (Professional Performance) Act 1995, the Council introduced its Performance Review Procedures designed to enhance its ability to detect and correct inappropriate standards in the delivery of clinical care by doctors.[53]

However, there is no sense in which the GMC acts as a co-ordinating body for the many other ways in which the profession regulates the performance of its members through the definition of standards, the monitoring and evaluation of performance against those standards, and the taking of corrective action where appropriate.

First, the setting of standards against which to measure clinical performance is very much in its infancy, but is generally regarded as the responsibility of the medical royal colleges and/or the specialist associations and societies. Some of those institutions are considerably more advanced than others in their development of relevant procedures. Senior officers of the Society of Cardiothoracic Surgeons, for example, are confident that it has the necessary database to support such procedures which 'should go some way to restoring public confidence' in the wake of the Bristol events.[54] It has, they claim, 'democratically assumed responsibility for quality control of individual surgical practices'—a new role for any specialist society within the UK.[55] However, the authors note that other specialities are in a much earlier stage of regulation development:

our specialty represents the tip of the iceberg in medical quality assurance, and
the major challenge will be determining realistic, measurable and auditable
outcomes for the other medical and surgical specialties, where poor outcomes
also occur but the process is less transparent.[56]

Given the pressures for change, this open political situation is likely
to pose problems for both medicine and the state.

As independent professional organisations, the royal colleges and
specialist societies are accountable to their members, not to the GMC
or to any other general regulation body. The speed at which they
respond to the need to establish standards of acceptable professional
practice (on which depend the other regulation stages of evaluation
and intervention) will vary in accordance with their internal organisational dynamics and their perception of the external demands.
Whether the state will be prepared to allow the required standards to
emerge on a specialty-by-specialty basis, unco-ordinated by any central
direction and according to a variable timescale, is questionable. Its
clear ambition announced in *A First Class Service* is that the National
Institute for Clinical Excellence should produce and disseminate
national clinical guidelines as part of its contribution to the development of best clinical practice.[57] Given this responsibility and its
avowed intent of working in partnership with the profession, NICE
may be obliged to take a leading role in ensuring that standards
development occurs.

As the originators of the standards which will underpin the regulation of medical performance, the royal colleges and specialist societies
are not unnaturally interested in the monitoring and evaluation of
clinical activity against those standards.[58] The Society of Cardiothoracic Surgeons maintains that 'measurement and interpretation should
be governed by the specialty'.[59] That being the case, there is then an
issue of how national standards, however they are determined, can be
incorporated into the existing procedures for local medical and clinical
audit and what institutional support is available to ensure that this
part of self-regulation works. In a candid moment, the combined
intellects of the BMA, Academy of Royal Colleges and Joint Consultants Committee (JCC) admitted that, over the past 20 years, clinical
and medical audit had 'largely failed' due mainly to the absence of
meaningful clinical outcome measurements.[60] Their view is supported
by independent research.[61] If those indicators are now going to be
produced, either by the royal colleges and specialist societies or, in a
separate initiative, by the JCC and the Academy of Royal Colleges,[62]
then the absence of a mechanism for ensuring their inclusion in local
clinical audit becomes starkly apparent. In this context the BMA
might well argue that its proposed system of consultant appraisal

based on peer review could be used to bridge the gap between national standards and local monitoring, though, as Johnson points out, 'to extend peer review to all specialties, even quinquennially in the first instance, would require a national initiative and financial support'.[63]

From the perspective of the medical profession, it is clear that the evolution of new mechanisms for performance monitoring is regarded as a lengthy process, involving a complex of institutions, upon which serious work, as opposed to token gestures, has only recently begun. Given the unstable political chemistry presently effervescing in the medicine/state relationship, such a view may prove to be, rightly or wrongly, catalytic. The state has already indicated its intention to remove the voluntary nature of current clinical performance monitoring. From 1999, all hospital doctors will be required to participate in a national audit programme appropriate to their specialty, endorsed by the new Commission for Health Improvement (CHI).[64] The logical next step is for the state to insist that doctors take part in local audit. In this respect it is significant that NICE's brief includes the development and dissemination of clinical audit methodologies[65] and that the new National Service Frameworks are intended to monitor performance against standards and outcomes[66]

If the monitoring of performance against particular standards reveals a deficiency, then the issue of intervention, the third type of regulation activity, becomes relevant. Which institution of medical self-regulation should take what corrective action in response to what type of performance deficiency? Given that systematic national standards and performance monitoring mechanisms have yet to be developed, either by the profession or the state, the politics of this knowledge control arena are, by definition, sketchy. Nonetheless, the interested parties in this emergent territory of self-regulation are clear enough.

Having worked long and hard to get its Performance Review Procedure accepted by both profession and state, it would be surprising if the GMC was not anxious that this should serve as the vehicle for intervention. The new procedure allows for a range of corrective actions to be taken once the nature of a doctor's poor performance is established, ranging from re-training to, eventually, removal from the register.[67] On the other hand, its potential scope is limited by its focus on not just poor performance, but on 'seriously deficient performance'. Others, and in particular the royal colleges, would argue that prevention is better than cure and that performance monitoring should be aiming at maintaining best practice rather than the identification of those who fall below a given standard.

In this respect, their burgeoning area of continuing medical education(CME) presents intervention through education as the appropriate answer to many of the issues prevalent in the performance regulatory arena. They have strong backing. The Chief Medical Officer placed CME at the heart of the triangle of forces when he argued that, whereas in previous years the legitimacy of a doctor's clinical competence was assured by the very fact of registration, now a 'more formal' and continuous system is required to assuage public doubts:

> The case for CME rests heavily on the concept of confidence: clinicians must command the confidence of the patients they treat; of the public as a whole; of the hospital managers to whom they are accountable for the quality of services to patients; and NHS managers who contract with hospitals on behalf of patients must have confidence in the quality of service they buy.[68]

But if CME is to act as a vehicle both for reassuring the public and for expanding the regulatory territory of the colleges, then it has to be consistent, comprehensive and mandatory, and seen to be so. At present it is doubtful whether the institutional conditions exist for the colleges to fulfil these conditions. As 12 fiercely independent bodies the colleges have so far evolved different systems of CME, achieved different levels of compliance amongst their members and introduced different sanctions for non-compliance with CME regulations. Those sanctions include: exclusion from being considered for merit awards and college committee membership (Royal College of Gynaecologists), loss of teacher status (Royal College of Ophthalmologists), and viewing a consultant without CME accreditation as a reason for the non-approval of training posts with which he/she is associated (Royal College of Physicians).[69] Such measures are unlikely to reassure the public since the logic of any regulatory intervention is that it must, if it is to be convincing, be linked to registration—i.e. fitness to practise. This, of course, brings us back to the GMC which, given its other registration functions, is the natural body to hold and administer a register of CME-accredited doctors.[70] Given that the colleges and the GMC have recently resolved the longstanding issue of the relationship between postgraduate accreditation and the Specialist Register, it is not wholly unrealistic to expect that a parallel political bargain could be struck over CME.

The Costs Of Change

Regardless of resolve, there is a point at which the medical profession's ability to manage change in its standard setting, evaluation, and intervention procedures is limited by the organisational and financial resources presently at its disposal. If it is to move beyond that point, it has to find either external support, or internal efficiencies, or both. It is likely that this is where medicine's dependence on the state for the privileges of self-regulation becomes manifest and where future political negotiations are likely to be concentrated.

For its part, the state is concerned to integrate medicine's self-regulation mechanisms within a broader system of clinical governance which forms part of the NHS's normal structure of public accountability. Trust chief executives, working through a designated senior clinician, now have responsibility for assuring the quality of clinical services provided by the trust.[71] Any improvements in self-regulation suggested by clinicians are therefore likely to be met with the condition that such changes be integrated with the trust's accountability systems. Indeed, the state's intention is pro-active in that clinical governance 'will provide a systematic framework that can be extended into the clinical community at all levels'.[72] Such an approach is likely to highlight the fact that the NHS has always had its own procedures for the regulation of the doctors it employs which have run parallel to but separate from those of the medical profession.[73] Rarely invoked and medically controlled, those procedures are either, in the less serious cases, a form of peer review or, where they could result in dismissal, are, in the words of the only formal study of their operation, 'legalistic, time-consuming, expensive and intimidating to those who might wish to report a problem or who might have something to say on the matter'.[74] At face value, therefore, their contribution to the maintenance of public confidence is likely to be limited.

Nonetheless, they constitute a battery of regulations on poor medical performance, situated within the line management of the NHS, which in the case of an individual doctor may lead to closer supervision, referral to an occupational health service, additional training, transfer to other duties, suspension and dismissal.[75] As management-led clinical governance moves forward, an important question for the medical profession is how to ensure that these and other NHS measures which impinge on the regulation of clinical practice (such as consultant job plans) fall within the medical and not the managerial sphere of influence. In this respect, positive intervention by medicine in local and national systems of accountability is unavoidable if it is to retain a formative role in the politics of self-regulation. Isolationism is not an option. It is significant that the Central Consultants and Specialists Committee (CCSC) of the BMA has recently issued guidance on how senior hospital doctors, clinical directors and medical directors should deal with concerns about the performance of consultants,[76] and is conducting further work on the role of clinical directors, their appraisal of consultants, the link between appraisal, consultant job plans and peer review, and the contribution to be made by external assessors.[77] Having for many years eschewed involvement in management, the profession is fast becoming aware that without it the resources for developing self-regulation may not be in its hands.

The state is no doubt aware that life in the NHS without the co-operation of doctors, in clinical governance as elsewhere, would be extremely difficult. For that reason *A First Class Service* contains much talk of partnership with the profession and of the contribution of doctors to the proposed national bodies for standard setting and monitoring. But at the same time the consultation paper is at pains to keep its political powder dry and to point out that, depending on progress in reducing the variations in clinical good practice, the powers of NICE and CHI may need to be strengthened in the future.[78] So the state is offering medicine, on the one hand, the opportunity to engage with the proposed structures of clinical governance to help make them work and, on the other, the threat that fresh powers will be brought to bear if this co-operation is not forthcoming. What it is not offering is new resources to support the arrangement: less the carrot-and-stick approach and more a two-sticks dilemma.

For medicine, harnessing the resources of the NHS to the needs of self-regulation is a necessary component of the management of change in that sphere, even if the price of this strategy is increased account-ability. But if medicine is to maximise the potential gains to be made from the present situation, it will need to improve the efficiency with which its élites operate, both in terms of their operation of more complex administrative systems of self-regulation and in terms of their approach to the rapidly changing relationship with the state. The existing set of loose alliances of GMC, royal colleges, BMA and JCC relies heavily on informal networks linked by key individuals to deal with the negotiation of both internal and external change. Such alliances may prove to be unwieldy vehicles for dealing with the stresses now apparent in the triangle of forces between medicine, civil society and the state. Thirty years ago, in her seminal work on the profession, Rosemary Stevens observed that 'many of the problems besetting the English professional associations of medicine have been not of authority in relation to the government but of their own interrelationships'.[79] Now that medicine has problems with the government as well, those divisions within the profession take on heightened significance.

Overcoming, or at least diminishing, the divisions within medicine, in order to achieve both a more efficient system of self-regulation and a unified political front, requires a re-ordering of the power hierarchy. If the needs of internal governance are to be given priority, then there has to be a clear accountability line between the regulation functions of standard setting, monitoring and evaluation, and intervention for each arena of knowledge control. This cannot be achieved unless institutions are prepared to forgo some of their current independence

in pursuit of the common professional good. Inevitably there will be
political costs: some institutions will gain and others will lose if
coherence is to be imposed on the presently fragmented nature of self-
regulation.

Conclusions

Whether the professional bodies of medicine have the political will, or
the capacity, to engage in what would amount to a radical reform of
their self-regulation system is unknown. Clearly there is awareness
among the élites of medicine that they have reached a political
Rubicon which somehow must be crossed. The CMO's Review Group,
on which those élites were represented, made it plain that 'the
professional responsibility to monitor the standards of colleagues'
professional performance needs to be reinforced for all doctors'.[80] And,
with regard to the whole gamut of self-regulation, the profession's
leading bodies admit that 'whilst there is a plethora of initiatives,
some less effective than others in ensuring self-regulation, there are
numerous "gaps" within the existing arrangements'.[81] Plugging those
gaps through individual institutional initiatives is likely to be a hit-
and-miss affair. Energised by the bracing air of the post-Bristol
climate, the Royal College of Physicians commissioned a study of its
functions which found that the College is perceived 'to have so far
failed to address urgent problems of self-regulation' and set out a long
list of recommendations for reform;[82] the Senate of Surgery of Great
Britain has recommended that surgeons should undergo professional
review every five years;[83] and the GMC has discussed possible forms
of revalidation for consultants and GPs.[84] However, the key question
of how these separate initiatives are to be co-ordinated so that they
constitute a single system of internal governance comprehensible to
the public has yet to be addressed.

In dealing with that question, the profession is not acting as an
isolated political entity. Its actions will impact on the triangle of
political forces between itself, civil society and the state in ways which
can be understood in terms of the political benefits which each accrues
as a result of participation in that triangle. Given the now highly
politicised nature of self-regulation, change in its internal institutional
and procedural arrangements can no longer take the form of a closed
professional activity, but is bound to engage the interest of society and
state—whether intentionally or not. In terms of the political benefits
which medicine gains from the triangle of forces, civil society will react
to such changes by increasing or decreasing its trust in the medical
profession and the state by the use of its clinical governance policy to
sustain, or to redefine, the nature of self-regulation. In the case of the

state, it is to be expected that its response will be constrained, at least to the extent that it acts rationally, by its need to maintain the viability of medicine both as a rationing agent and the instrument for the delivery of its citizens' healthcare rights. It cannot afford to throw away the baby with the bathwater. In the case of society, no such calculation is present and it is here that the essential volatility of the situation lies and hence the risk to the stability of the triangle of forces as a whole.

This is new political territory for both medicine and the state. For the first 40 years of the NHS the hegemony of the medical profession went unchallenged. Then, when it was challenged by the reforms of the internal market, any possibility that these would have a real impact on medicine's essential power base, the control of knowledge, was removed by the automatic exclusion of medical self-regulation from the policy debate surrounding the reforms. By this action the challenge was emasculated, the ability of the medical profession to maintain its own separate sphere of governance within the NHS was preserved, and in due course the imperatives of the triangle of forces reasserted themselves. What has altered the balance of forces between medicine, civil society and the state significantly, and thrust self-regulation blinking into the political daylight, is not so much the state's decision to enter the heartland of medical power through the assumption of responsibility for clinical governance, as the public's newly awakened awareness that it can no longer trust the medical profession to deliver health care of an appropriate quality. As the state is presumably aware, whilst societal concern is currently directed at the medical profession, a failure by medicine convincingly to reform its system of self-regulation combined with the state's prominent claim to have assumed the mantle of clinical governance must make the state the public's next target.

The political logic of the situation would therefore suggest that it is in the interest of both medicine and the state to embrace a new form of corporatism. Unlike that which characterised the previous concordat, where medicine dominated,[85] this would engage both medicine and state as equal partners in a contractual arrangement designed to maintain the political benefits which historically each has gained from the triangle of political forces, but on a new basis. The key to the new contract would be a joint approach to the politics of self-regulation whereby the state enabled the medical profession to develop a new system of internal governance on condition that this approach (a) was acceptable to society and (b) incorporated the principle of public accountability as enshrined in the clinical governance policy. Using heavy political advice, reinforced by reserve legislative muscle, the state's role would be to help define the new power relationships required within medicine in order to rationalise the present fragmented system of self-regulation and judiciously release resources as progress was achieved. Medicine, meanwhile, would be obliged to hone its informal system of conflict resolution. However, whether logic will prevail is dependent on public opinion, that eternal unknown, which no politician can ignore.

The General Medical Council and Professional Self-Regulation

Meg Stacey

The General Medical Council (GMC) was set up by Act of Parliament in 1858 to ensure the public could trust any doctor who was registered with it: that was the profession's promise to the state. A statutory body, it was nevertheless set up on the principle of self-regulation, that is to say the Council was entirely in the profession's hands, being financed then as now by the profession itself. This status was the culmination of a long struggle, achieved only after several bills put before parliament had failed.

In the first half of the nineteenth century there were many kinds of healers. The allopaths, who have now become our biomedical practitioners, were only one of that wide range. It was they who gained this special status. The 1858 Act did not stop other healers from practising, but no other healers could call themselves 'registered medical practitioners'. The establishment of the GMC gave the registered allopathic healers great advantages over the others. The earning power of registered practitioners improved greatly compared with what it had been before the GMC was established and in comparison with other healers. Being registered with the Council gave practitioners a monopoly as advisers to the state (no other practitioners could, for example, get a job in the armed forces or in a government department).

For many years this bargain between the state and the medical profession went virtually unchallenged. The state and the GMC worked closely together. It suited both to avoid any discussion in parliament of the GMC.[1] When, in 1976, I was appointed to sit on the GMC as a 'lay' member (i.e. not medically qualified) few people were aware of what the Council did or how it did it. Indeed the General Medical Council and the British Medical Association (BMA) were—and still are—often confused. The GMC, as already noted, is a statutory body with a duty to regulate the profession in the interests of the public. The BMA, on the other hand, is the doctors' trade union and is affiliated to the TUC. The BMA does concern itself with ethical matters, but its prime purpose is to protect the profession.

In 1976 the GMC was a remote and shadowy body to the bulk of doctors as well as their patients. Doctors and the public were aware that the Council could strike a doctor off the register. This awareness came largely from cases the press deemed newsworthy, usually because of some sexual transgression. Otherwise the GMC rarely came into the public eye. However, since the 'Bristol case' in 1999—when surgeons were disciplined as a result of their treatment of children undergoing heart surgery and the high death rates which resulted —this has changed. As the editor of the *BMJ* put it: 'All changed, changed utterly'.[2] There is high awareness of the risks involved in modern medical treatment (as well as of the marvels it can perform) and much more doubt about whether doctors can be trusted to regulate themselves.

This chapter will illustrate the pros and cons of professional self-regulation (PSR) in the particular case of the GMC, asking whether it is an adequate way of regulating medicine. The discussion will be based on my experiences as a lay member of the GMC from 1976 to 1983 and upon research I did after my term of office was completed. This research was published in 1992[3] but I have kept an eye on developments since then. The Council as it now exists is different in many ways from the Council I joined nearly a quarter of a century ago, as I will demonstrate. Before I go into those details, however, I shall say something about the regulation of occupations and where self-regulation fits in.

Why Only Professional *Self-regulation?*

All occupations can make a case for self-regulation as follows:

No one knows better than the worker involved what it means to do a job, under what conditions it is possible to do that job properly—in the workplace and in terms of the rewards received. The worker knows best when the job is being, or has been, done properly; anyway it is in the workers' interests to do a good job to gain trust, work opportunities and advancement.

It is inferred that the interests of the buyers of labour coincide with those of the workers. However, in the vast majority of occupations these arguments are given no credence. There seems to be agreement that it would lead to chaos. After all, a disciplined workforce is required; the managers and directors know what output they want; the workers must do what they are told; they can't be trusted; their work must be inspected and overseen.

But a special case is made by the professions who argue in the following way.

Our work is highly individualistic, each person is unique, each case different. Furthermore, given the esoteric nature of the knowledge and the long training required, only insiders can possibly know how the work should be done or regulated. However, aware that ours is a job which may enhance or reduce a client's life and very being, we accept a special moral obligation to be trustworthy and to support the general good of society by being honourable and upright citizens.

The Regulative Bargain

Where the claim to professional status is successful, as it was in the case of medicine, a 'regulative bargain'[4] is struck between the representatives of the organised occupation and agents of the state whereby the privilege of self-regulation is given in return for the promise of ensuring good service. This is the culmination of the 'professional project'.[5] The professional project refers to the organised activities of individuals who come together for the purpose of achieving recognition for their occupation. It is the leaders of this organised collectivity who make the bargain and have the responsibility to maintain it. *Professionals* are the individual practitioners who are permitted to bear the title, while *a profession* refers to the collectivity of organised practitioners.

The regulative bargain gives privileges to professionals over all other occupations: privileges such as autonomy in the workplace; a near monopoly of the market; the facility to regulate terms and conditions of work. Professionals and their organisations nevertheless remain subject to the rule of law. In return for these outstanding privileges professionals promise—through the leaders of the profession—that all those who carry the title shall be competent and trustworthy, such that they may be approached with confidence by potential clients, who inevitably lack specialist knowledge. The professions promise that they will regulate themselves to this end. This last involves ensuring that only those who are appropriately trained and educated may enter the profession; further, that any who deviate from these standards shall be disciplined and removed from the profession if necessary.[6]

Self-regulation is perhaps *the* hallmark of a profession, but cultural aspects are also important. 'Individuals strive more or less consciously, more or less overtly, to distinguish themselves from their friends and competitors; presenting themselves as having the standing, the knowledge, the skill, the demeanour appropriate to a vet, a midwife, a barrister or a [doctor].' Equivalent efforts are made at the level of the practice or firm and of the professional association.[7]

In practice 'pure self-regulation' is rarely found. Internationally there is a range from those where professions are independent of the state, as in the US, through those which are state-sanctioned but self-regulating, as in the UK, to those which are directly state-run, as in continental Europe. Until recently much research (including mine) has had an Anglo-Saxon bias. The variations in the external/internal mix are enlightening and historical in origin.[8] A comparison of changes over time is also interesting, as will emerge.

The Regulatory Tasks

Whoever does the regulating, there are certain tasks to be performed. Allsop and Mulcahy, expanding on Moran and Wood,[9] have listed them as follows:

1 Control of market entry and exit

2 Control of competitive practices

3 Control of market organisation

4 Control of remuneration

5 Ensuring safety.

While regulation has a great deal to do with the market, it also 'involves issues of good practice, accountability, efficiency and ethics'.[10] Whoever regulates and howsoever they do it, moral values and moral choices are involved.[11]

The Case Of The GMC

Sir Donald Irvine, the current President of the GMC, has articulated its tasks as follows.

1 To keep a register of those doctors it has licensed as competent to practise in the UK

2 To set general standards of medical practice

3 To determine the nature of university-based medical education; to ensure implementation; and to co-ordinate all stages of medical education

4 To deal with dysfunctional doctors whose registration has been called into question.[12]

These points cover items 1 and 5 on Allsop and Mulcahy's list and to some extent item 2.

The register, with which Sir Donald's list begins and ends, is the main instrument through which the GMC fulfils the first task. The register is a powerful instrument, since the law requires all doctors to be registered before they may practise. The GMC controls entry to the register by deciding what qualifications are necessary for registration—Sir Donald's point 3; it can remove practitioners from the register temporarily or permanently when they are deemed to have become unfit to practise, and (nowadays) may put conditions on a doctor's registration (point 4).

The Council works through committees that deal with each aspect of its work. The Education Committee works with the medical schools to determine the qualifications necessary for entry to the register. Disciplinary issues, when a question arises as to whether a doctor is fit to continue to practise, are dealt with by two committees, namely the Preliminary Proceedings Committee (PPC) and the Professional Conduct Committee (PCC). Complaints or reports received by the Council are initially sifted to see if they fall within the Council's jurisdiction. If so, they are passed to the PPC which decides whether there is a *prima facie* case to answer; if there is, the case is passed to the PCC which then undertakes a full inquiry as to the practitioner's continued fitness to practise. This is done in a judicial manner with a high standard of proof required and a legal adviser to help the committee, which is composed mostly of doctors but includes some lay people.

Until the 1978 Medical Act, all cases of suspected fitness to practise had to go down that route. Since 1978, where the alleged unfitness is thought to be caused by ill health (physical or mental and including alcohol and drug addiction), the case is dealt with by the Health Committee. Thus at the end of the 1970s there were three main sets of procedures concerned with entry to and exit from the Register.

The Legitimacy Of The Council

Given professional self-regulation, the Council can only wield the power which statutory control of the Register gives it so long as its legitimacy is recognized by the bulk of medical practitioners and the profession remains united. In the late 1960s and early 1970s, the unity of the profession and the legitimacy of the GMC were nearly lost. The catalyst for the professional revolt of those years was the introduction—or imposition as many doctors saw it—of an annual retention fee to remain on the register. Hitherto, the fee the doctors paid when they first qualified lasted them a lifetime.

Even before the annual fee was suggested, there had been discontent with a Council seen as top-heavy with elderly men from universities, royal colleges and London hospitals. The Council was failing to represent NHS consultants and specialists; it had never had a proportionate representation of GPs; and it included no junior hospital doctors. That it also lacked doctors who had qualified overseas was not much noticed then. Nor was the under-representation of women. There were only three women on the Council in 1976 out of a total of 46 and only one of us medically qualified.

That upheaval led to the 1978 Medical Act which doubled the size of the Council and gave a majority to elected over appointed members (that is, members appointed by royal colleges and universities). Reforms that the old Council had wanted, such as the introduction of the Health Committee (mentioned above) to deal more humanely with sick and addicted doctors, were included in the legislation. The 1978 reforms were profession-led and addressed problems identified by medical people. Among other things the proportion of lay members was reduced, although their absolute number was increased.

Public Interest And Anxiety Increases

As the 1980s opened and the provisions of the 1978 Act were working their way through the Council's activities, further criticisms began to be made. These came from outside the profession. The virtual monopoly accorded to the professions did not chime well with the free-market ideology of the Thatcher government. Professions ceased to be sacrosanct. Medicine was now seen as a trade like any other commercial activity. Patient pressure groups, increasingly knowledgeable about medicine and healthcare organisation, encouraged patients to be critical and take action when they felt things were not right. Not all lay members of the GMC were 'more medical than the medics' as at one time they had seemed to be. The patients were beginning to have a voice.

In 1982 the GMC disciplined one Dr Archer who had allegedly not attended properly to a sick child, Alfie Winn. Alfie subsequently died. The way the GMC handled this case set up a chain of consequences. Alfie was the mascot of the West Ham United Football Club and lived in the constituency of Nigel Spearing MP. The committee who heard the case found the charges against Dr Archer proved: that he had not referred Alfie for the specialist attention he needed and had been discourteous to Alfie's parents. The committee did not consider this amounted to serious professional misconduct (SPM: the conclusion necessary to remove a person from the register) and simply admonished Dr Archer. To Alfie's mother and to Spearing this seemed an inadequate outcome.

Spearing came to believe that a verdict of SPM might have been inappropriate but that an admonition was undoubtedly insufficient. He developed a case for a second and lesser charge of *unacceptable professional conduct*. The New Zealand Council already had such a two-tier system. In 1984 Nigel Spearing introduced the first of a series of bills to provide a two-tier system for the GMC. The latter did not like parliamentary interference, did not like the idea of two tiers, but realised that it was under serious scrutiny and set about working to forestall the attacks. Their determination was no doubt sharpened by a number of further scandals and exposures.[13]

The media was now on the trail. In the television programme *That's Life* Esther Rantzen exposed the private practice of a Dr Frempong who used laser surgery when he was not competent to do so and damaged many patients who had to go to other doctors to be repaired. These doctors, however, did not report Frempong as incompetent. Duncan Campbell, investigative journalist, exposed Drs. Sharp and Sultan who were conning AIDS patients with promises of a cure. Again, although other doctors knew about this malpractice, they did not report it. Increasingly, it became apparent that self-regulation was not regulating in the interests of the patients and public.

In those days members of the medical profession were advised by the GMC not to tell on each other. This ruling derived from the profession's need to keep medical practitioners united, necessary for PSR to work. However, as Mrs Jean Robinson, an outspoken lay member, has argued, this led to a culture of secrecy and deceit in so far as serious malpractice cases were not reported. In 1983 the advice began to be modified. Mrs Robinson worked hard to get the original wording changed.[14] Finally the ruling was completely reversed.

In *Good Medical Practice*,[15] the GMC spells out the duties of a doctor. This makes quite clear that a practitioner who has evidence that another is incompetent to practise for whatever reason, or is not practising ethically, has a responsibility to take action. In the section headed 'Your duty to protect all patients', paragraph 23 reads: 'You must protect patients when you believe that a doctor's or other colleague's health, conduct or performance is a threat to them.' Paragraph 24 then spells out details of how to do this, concluding: 'The safety of patients must come first at all times.'[16] This represents a major change in practice and culture. How far this new understanding has yet spread throughout the profession is unclear. No one ever likes to shop a colleague, even with strong official guidance to do so. However, the responsibility is now clear: a doctor knowing about and failing to report a malfunctioning colleague may be disciplined by the GMC.

Dealing With Incompetent Doctors

The GMC had always been slow to examine the clinical aspects of complaints and reluctant to accept that serious incompetence amounted to SPM.[17] The doctrine of clinical autonomy, a cherished component of the professional project, claimed that only the doctor in attendance could know what was proper to be done for a patient. If what s/he did was called to account, then only persons in the same specialty could judge. Although members of the GMC's disciplinary committees were all medically qualified, with a minority of lay persons, and relevant specialists were always in attendance, the GMC had over the years been extremely reluctant to judge clinical competence to practise. However, my research also showed that during the 1980s more clinical competence cases began to be referred from the PPC to the PCC. Alfie's case was one such.

The GMC was becoming aware that it had to be more clearly seen to be doing its job of protecting the public. The resolution of its investigations as to how best to forestall legislation such as Nigel Spearing wanted was to propose a new disciplinary procedure relating to *professional performance*. This, the Council argued, would make it possible to discipline doctors whose general performance was poor, and who consistently under-performed. Under-performance might arise because a doctor had let her/his medical knowledge and skills fall behind the fast-changing scene, s/he might have become slipshod in behaviour, not attending to patients when called, and might also be behaving consistently rudely and inappropriately. Such a doctor might not be, or not yet, caught in a serious fault of the kind that would bring her/him before the PCC.

This author still is unable to understand why the Council needed new powers for this. Does not seriously poor performance amount to serious professional misconduct? Nor was I alone in this. However, finally parliamentary time was requested to legislate for new procedures. The delay was partly because of the GMC's need to consult with all the other bodies involved one way and another in medical regulation and its need to keep the profession as a whole behind it. Also, the Council was afraid to ask for legislation in the strongly anti-professional atmosphere which Thatcher had created, being afraid it might get more that it had bargained for. The Council has an excellent record of achieving legislation which is broadly along the lines of whatever compromises it has itself come to within the profession. Legislation was finally passed in 1995; the professional performance procedures are now in place, some 12 years after they began to be thought about. The very considerable task of applying them in practice is now in hand.[18]

Bristol may be the dramatic divider, but reforms were well underway when Sir Donald Irvine became President of the Council in 1995, the first general practitioner to hold that office and a sign in itself of the changing times. 1995 was also the year when the first edition of *Good Medical Practice*[19] was published. Sir Donald, as chairman of the GMC standards committee, had played an important part in its development.

His belief in good practice and the need to be seen to act to maintain standards was, I believe, what led him to handle the 'Bristol case' as he did. Ironically, in the short run, more doctors than ever before now see the GMC as punitive. For the public, that case took the lid off unsatisfactory practices, revealing what a few had known about, many more suspected, but none had been able to see so clearly or, if they saw, had adequate means to deal with. In the short term the upshot appears to have increased public suspicion of the Council and of the medical profession in general.

What Was The Bristol Case?

The Bristol case was an inquiry by the GMC into the behaviour of three doctors (two surgeons and a chief executive) in relation to the deaths of 29 babies and young children who had had elective surgery at the Bristol Royal Infirmary. All three doctors were found guilty of SPM: James Wisheart, a former senior surgeon and medical director at Bristol, was struck off the medical register; another surgeon, Janardan Dhasmana, was allowed to remain registered but banned from doing paediatric surgery for three years; Dr John Roylance, former chief executive of United Bristol Health Care Trust, was struck off. This last signalled that managerial as well as clinical skills were up for sanction. Janardan Dhasmana and James Wisheart had been warned that their death rates were too high. John Roylance knew about the complaints but did not act.

The case caught the attention of patients, the public and doctors as none before. The events were dramatic and tragic. Not only was the surgery below par, but the risks had not been properly spelled out. This was not surgery to save life in immediate danger but to improve the quality (and hopefully length) of life. In addition to the apparently unnecessary deaths and damage which the little ones suffered, the length of time that the mistakes had been going on appalled everyone.

The whistle had been blown in 1990 by Dr Stephen Bolsin, an anaesthetist at the hospital. He 'suffered the traditional fate of whistleblowers, ostracism and collapse in earnings'[20] and ultimately left the country to practise in Australia. After the verdicts were announced, six other Bristol doctors (Gianni Angelini, professor of cardiac surgery, Andy Black, Sheila Willats and Ian Davies, anaesthetists, Alan Bryan, surgeon and Peter Wilde, radiologist) pointed out that they had tried to initiate action, blaming the regulative bodies and the government for failing to act.

From some medical practitioners' points of view there was a sense of undue harshness—that heart surgery is always risky; that the conditions were congenital; that the practitioner had gone back to a centre of excellence to train further when he felt his record was perhaps not good enough. Frank Dobson, the Secretary of State—

rather out of turn—joined the bereaved parents in saying he thought Dhasmana should also have been struck off.

The whole tragedy raised many more points about the regulation of medicine than the GMC is empowered by law to deal with and many more children died or were damaged than were included in the hearing. These features led to frustration among the parents. Indeed the GMC recognized its limitations.[21]

Is The Government Taking Over Medical Regulation?

From the 1980s, as I have indicated above, government began to pay attention to self-regulation. Before the Bristol case broke the government had already become pro-active. While some of the problems arose from within the GMC with its inherited protective practices and its reactive culture, others arose from the multiplicity of ancient medical institutions, each responsible for bits of the regulatory process. Crucially, yet other problems derived from the failure over 50 years to relate the regulation of the NHS to professional self-regulation.

Two command papers from the Department of Health signal the government's felt need to take action: *The New NHS: Modern, Dependable* and *A First Class Service: Quality in the New NHS*.[22] The government has established a National Institute for Clinical Excellence (NICE) to work on clinical guidelines and their application within the NHS. Immediately after the GMC verdicts came out and after the near riots outside the GMC headquarters, the government set up a public inquiry. It is now sitting with the lawyer Ian Kennedy in the chair, who was the first on a very public platform (the Reith lectures) to draw attention to failures in medical regulation. Whereas the GMC was restricted to the part played by doctors, the Kennedy inquiry in contrast has a wide brief to look at all the surrounding features and players involved. Certainly, the government has accepted responsibility in new ways. The result is a plethora of new bodies.[23]

The Medical Response

These have been added to by activity among the old medical bodies (such as the royal colleges) aimed to defend PSR and to show that medical self-regulation can work. For example, the Royal College of Surgeons of England and the Society of Cardiothoracic Surgeons will provide a 'rapid response group' so that a member of the College council and a senior thoracic surgeon can be on site within 48 hours when trouble is signalled.[24] Advice and guidance on clinical matters are relatively new ideas in most specialties (anaesthetics and obstetrics being honourable exceptions). 'Interference' in the clinical autonomy of colleagues was previously unthinkable. The rapid response group will, if it works well, enhance the prestige of the cardiothoracic surgeons as well as saving patient life and improving well-being.

What Will Be The Effect On The GMC And On Medical Self-regulation?

There is no doubt that the GMC took a risk in hearing this case. The inquiry was long; it lasted over 65 days and cost £2.2 million. It was hard and harrowing: many were the medical and legal challenges, long the hours and days worked. In a sense it was a gamble for the life of the GMC and medical self-regulation overall. Undoubtedly events had reached a situation in which, without action, self-regulation would be lost by default. If PSR could not be shown to work in the conditions of modern medicine, medical regulation would be taken from medical practitioners.

Are the reforms 'too little too late'? Should the Council not have listened more attentively to its critics, some from 15 years ago and earlier?[25] Can PSR ever work? What are the hazards of the other options? Does the government really want to take over the whole of the complex task, with its high costs (currently paid for by the profession) and including the question of maintaining legitimacy which now lies with the GMC and all the other medical regulatory bodies?

Two incompatible ways have been suggested whereby the case for PSR may prevail. One is putting on a good front, the second, reform for real. The first is to follow the route which Brandt[26] thinks professionalisation has already taken, that is, 'a transformation from a "group-in-itself" to a "group-for-itself" while simultaneously *appearing* as a "group-for-others"' (my emphasis). That is, doing a competent public relations job so that, whatever happens, the profession *appears* trustworthy. Such a project might last for a while, but in the end would be exposed. All of the people cannot be kidded all of the time—as Bristol showed.

There is a hint of the good public relations approach in the title of an article 'Making self-regulation credible'. Its content, however, suggests a more serious intent and is directed at advising doctors to get their act together quickly, because 'patients need to know that they will be safe when hospital treatment is necessary'.[27] In so doing the article smacks more of the second view, that PSR should be made to work in the terms of the regulative bargain.

In 1996 I said that reform was needed to avoid the trap of delusions which lead regulators to *mean well but do badly*, as was certainly the case when I sat on the GMC. 'External help must be invited and self-regulation must be publicly and regularly accountable.'[28] The GMC has taken on board its need for external advice and the government is paying attention to its accountability.

Pure PSR has always been a myth. The balance of external and internal control has varied from country to country. In Britain today the balance has shifted a bit towards external governmental control, through the NHS reforms and new institutions such as NICE, but that is not all. The medical profession now seems intent upon regulating pro-actively. Both profession and government are paying more attention to the local level and its relation to national bodies such as the GMC and the royal colleges.

In less than 25 years the Council has been quite radically changed. In 1976 there were three lay members out of a total of 46. Since 1997 lay people have made up a quarter of the 104-strong Council. They are not elected but many are nominated by bodies to which they may refer. Lay people are involved in the performance procedures, although not on a basis fully equal with the professionals. The duties of a doctor have been clearly spelled out so that both doctors and patients may be clear about what is expected. The Council is much more pro-active in maintaining standards in clinical practice than when I was first a lay member, when only the grossest of cases ever came before it. Klein[29] has suggested that all the doubts about the GMC's commitment to the public have now been dispelled.

Many members of the public still have doubts. We wait to see whether these will be dispelled as the years pass. We must also wait to see whether the legitimacy of the GMC can be maintained in its new, more rigorous, form. Within the present Council the omens are good. In the face of a challenge, Sir Donald was re-elected President in 1999. The next elections to Council will show which way the voting rank and file wish to go. Furthermore, the tasks facing the profession as a whole are many and complex. Whatever happens, British medicine and PSR will never be the same again.

Self-Regulation and the
Role of the General Medical Council

James Johnson

It is ironic that when the General Medical Council strikes a doctor off the medical register in a highly publicised case, the event is closely followed by a chorus of vituperation in the press to the effect that there is now clear proof that the profession can no longer regulate itself. Why should this be? The fact that the doctor has been disciplined is clear evidence that the profession *is* regulating itself, but a close analysis of the media stories shows their concern to be centred around those patients who were harmed before the time when the doctor was called to account. There is clearly a desire for a system which disciplines doctors at a much earlier stage—before so much damage has been done— and preferably before any damage has been done at all. Such a hope may not be realistic. It may not even be remotely possible— though few could question its desirability.

For its part, the profession is baffled and wounded by the constant attacks made on it. The number of doctor/patient transactions which take place annually in the NHS runs into millions; the number of individual decisions which doctors make about patients and their treatment is uncountable, so how often can a doctor be expected to get it right? The positive side of medicine constantly emphasises the hi-tech miracles that can be performed. The same newspapers that call for draconian punishments for erring doctors will run on the next page a story of artificial hearts, or transplantation of limbs, resulting in public expectations of what medicine can provide which are totally unrealistic. Doctors and ministers are their own worst enemies in this respect. Medics revel in publicity for advances in medicine, and media attention for the research of an individual or an institution is often a means of attracting funds. Ministers, always aware that they can never really win with the NHS, also act to build up patients' expectations—through patients' charters and the like—beyond anything that the NHS can hope to achieve. No-one is prepared to give the honest view, which is that biological systems show an infinite variability, not found in television sets or jumbo jets; that at the end of the twentieth century diagnosis is often no more than an educated guess based on physical findings and medical tests, the results of which are frequently contradictory; and that success in technical procedures is frustrated every bit as much by adverse patient variations (such as obesity or other co-morbidity) as by lack of manual dexterity or knowledge on the part of the doctor.

So how often can the doctor get it right—nine times out of ten, 99 times out of 100? Whatever the figure, it is clearly finite. In a region where the cervical screening 'mistakes' were said to be a cause for concern, the allegation was made on the basis of an error rate of 0.1 per cent in more than 90,000 specimens. The public needs to understand that no system in the world will prevent doctors from making occasional mistakes, and that an organisation the size of the NHS will always have incidents which it would rather forget. The sheer scale of the organisation makes this inevitable.

But realism must not be an excuse for complacency. The General Medical Council generally works well and fairly. It cannot be blamed for failures which have not been drawn to its attention, though it could speed up its processes when this has happened. Its main failing in the context of self-regulation (and this is not a criticism) is that it is a central body working out of London. It does not have a peripheral arm: there are no regional offices, let alone a representative in each hospital or doctor's surgery. So what is needed is an explicit partnership between the profession and the GMC to roll out effective self-regulation into the workplace. This is the way to identify under-performing doctors earlier, and hopefully before patients have been harmed. There is a need for a culture change in British medicine to emphasise that quality and self-regulation—for the two go hand-in-hand—are the business of every doctor, not just the regulatory body (GMC) and the royal colleges. But this culture change must be based on matters which are more tangible, and have more substance, than good intentions. I would propose four areas where changes of substance need to be made to permit self-regulation to not only police the profession, but to encourage a quantum leap in standards across the board.

1. Outcome Data

Outcomes in medicine vary enormously, from hard and unarguable facts (e.g. the percentage of patients who die within 30 days of a particular operation), to subjective opinions (the measurable effects of psychotherapy on a range of behavioural problems), to public health issues (the effect of a campaign to provide sex education and free contraception on teenage pregnancy rates), to wider epidemiological issues (the ability of a national service framework to affect the mortality and morbidity of a population from coronary heart disease).

The common thread is the dearth of information available to allow individual doctors or teams to compare their own outcomes with those of the NHS as a whole. If doctors have nothing to use as comparators for their own results, it will seem a fairly pointless exercise to collect these results, and those who do will be none the wiser. Ironically, the specialty with the best outcome data for work across the whole of the NHS is cardiac surgery. This specialty is characterised by a relatively small number of different procedures, being carried out in relatively few hospitals by a relatively small number of surgeons —factors which make data collection easy. As a result, cardiac surgeons can compare their own results with those of colleagues. The result of this ability, however, has not been a happy one for the specialty, as recent events have shown, and can hardly be seen as an incentive for others to do likewise. But it is important not to be deflected from what is an important initiative. The NHS desperately needs outcome data. The Academy of Medical Royal Colleges is currently encouraging all its members and the specialty associations to engage in a rolling programme of data collection, and the Department of Health is providing financial support.

It is difficult to overemphasise the need for such action. If a surgeon knows that (say) 95 per cent of surgeons performing a particular operation have a mortality 30 days after surgery of between two and five per cent, that surgeon can compare his own performance with his peers. Doctors with results falling short of the norms would wish to take urgent action to improve the results. Where the outcome was an unacceptable mortality, for instance, it might be necessary for the clinician concerned, together with the clinical and medical director, to decide to stop performing the operation or procedure until corrective action could be taken. Similarly, those doctors with results better than the norm could serve as exemplars from which the NHS as a whole could learn how to improve performance.

Once national outcomes were known, the information systems of a hospital or a group practice could churn out the relevant data for its own professionals. There would be no question therefore of persuading doctors to come to audit; the 'machine' would produce and update the information, and doctors and their managers could have before them data which demonstrated without any shadow of a doubt whether the results of their department were acceptable in the context of the NHS as a whole.

It is sometimes said that outcome data is available from the medical literature, but this is rarely the case. Textbooks quote figures for outcomes based on papers written by doctors who wish to tell colleagues about their excellent results. On this basis the recurrence rate after primary repair of an inguinal hernia is generally quoted as being about five per cent. It is probable that the recurrence rate for most surgeons and their junior staff is considerably higher than this. We simply do not know, and therefore find it difficult to criticise colleagues for poor technique in this operation, because we have nothing with which to compare their results.

In areas where hard *outcomes* are difficult to find, doctors must be content with auditing *process*. A unit could compare its own work with a basket of process measures agreed by the NHS as a whole. One measure might be the length of time to get a hospital appointment after referral by a GP with a particular condition. The caveat here is that the processes compared must have genuine importance to patients or be based on scientific evidence. Too often process measures are based on some political fad (being spoken to by the 'hello nurse' in an accident and emergency department) and have little relevance to what matters to patients (how long they will have to wait before they see a doctor).

Outcome measures would make the GMC's task much simpler. The difficulty with the current performance process is how to tell whether a doctor is under-performing or whether he is a fairly average example of a doctor in his specialty. Outcome data would clarify that.

2. Peer Review And Appraisal

Both the British Medical Association and the Academy of Medical Royal Colleges have concluded that the time is right to introduce an appraisal system which looks both at the role of the individual and of the department or organisation, and which is clearly rooted in peer review. It would be wholly meaningless for the clinical aspects of doctors' work to be judged by lay managers or even by doctors from different specialties. They would simply not have the knowledge or technical expertise to decide whether a doctor or his service was adequate and satisfactory, or whether it fell below the line of accept-ability. Admittedly, hard outcome data would help, but, as stated above, it is seldom available and a comprehensive set of outcome data is many years away. Systems have been pioneered in thoracic medicine (and are about to be piloted in diabetes) for a team from one unit to visit and make an extended assessment of both the capacity and capability of the doctor in a second unit, and the facilities, equipment, staffing levels, and so on in a second unit, in a different hospital doing broadly similar work. Such a project, if extended to all specialties and sub-specialties, could be ambitious and organisationally complex, but at the end of the day it is the only way to guarantee to the public that professional and technical standards are up to scratch. The thoracic physicians have found the system to be of value in maintaining standards, and in driving management to invest in proper staffing and equipment. Similarly the evidence provided by external peer review could be clear and factual evidence to the hospital clinical governance committee, to the Commission for Health Improvement and to the General Medical Council of the prevailing standards of individual doctors in the context of the hospital in which they work, and would make the assessment of doctors whose performance is questioned much more straightforward. It is difficult to overemphasise to the public the difficulties faced by the hospitals and the GMC when investigating alleged under-performance or incompetence in the absence of any hard facts.

I have stated that a system of external peer review would be ambitious and organisationally complex. It would also be expensive. The costs lie not only in the expense of the visit—travel, accommodation and so on—but in the opportunity costs of clinical work not done by those preparing to be reviewed, and by the reviewers. A balance must be struck between the time doctors spend reviewing each other and the time spent treating patients, between the frequency of the reviews (ideally annually) and what the NHS can afford (perhaps every five or even ten years to begin with).

3. Revalidation

The General Medical Council is looking at what is meant by 'maintaining a register'. Recently, specialist registration has been added to general or basic registration—though there is as yet no equivalent mechanism to identify those doctors who have completed training in general practice. Standards of entry to the specialist register are high and rigorous. But how can the public know that a doctor who conformed to exacting standards at the time of obtaining a certificate of completion of specialist training (CCST) continues to conform ten or 20 years later? Revalidation would be a method of assessment (in its broadest sense) which would demonstrate that standards are maintained. The idea has obtained widespread support in principle, but presents formidable (though not insuperable) problems to implement. Most significant of these is: what happens when revalidation identifies a problem? The GMC has in the last few years set up a series of procedures aimed at identifying problems where remedial action can put the matter right. These 'performance procedures' are a welcome addition to the older and better known disciplinary procedures used to deal with medical 'high crimes and misdemeanours' in which a guilty verdict means suspension or erasure from the register, with consequential loss of livelihood. While revalidation might identify such matters, it seems likely that it would more usually highlight areas of performance which are below par but capable of improvement with appropriate corrective action. There seems therefore to be a link between any system of revalidation and the new performance procedures. The royal colleges and specialist societies (who would be instrumental in organising external peer review) might also take on the role of rehabilitation or salvage of the under-performing doctor, by arranging a package of re-training for individual practitioners. The postgraduate deans might also extend their remit to this group of doctors. It is likely that the practical problems will be resolved and that revalidation will be added to the GMC's armamentarium within the next few years.

4. Continuing Professional Development (CPD)

For some years now the medical royal colleges have monitored the continuing professional development of their members and fellows by a system of credits for different educational activities. The colleges will soon be able to produce lists of those of their members who have fulfilled the requirements of CPD. Some colleges will produce and may well publish these lists, and others will follow. They will provide tangible evidence that doctors on the lists have taken adequate steps to keep up-to-date and to maintain their knowledge base—and will provide the public with further evidence of continuing ability to practise.

The final area which I wish to explore is the intensity of doctors' work. This may seem irrelevant to a discussion of self-regulation and the General Medical Council, but it has a direct bearing on the issue. The NHS's astonishing value for money—undoubtedly the envy of the governments of developed countries—is due in part to low wages across the service, in part to a no-nonsense, no frills approach to healthcare, and in part to a very heavy caseload and intensity of working for doctors and other health professionals. While the public is largely unconcerned about wages, the no-frills approach and the intensity of working increasingly causes problems in an increasingly consumerist society. The no-frills approach with its waiting lists, queues, poor hospital food and dormitory accommodation for in-patients is probably the principle reason why patients opt for private medicine, rather than because of concerns about professional care.

And the high intensity of work simply means less time for a doctor to spend with each patient, leading to poor communication and short-cuts in clinical care. The Health Ombudsman regularly publishes *Investigations Completed*, reports of cases brought before him, and, in a great many of the commonest complaints referred to him, lack of time leading to poor communication can be found at the root of the problem.

The GMC's own advice to doctors, though excellent in theory, simply could not be followed in practice without reducing the size of (say) hospital clinics and operating lists by a very significant amount. The result of this would be escalating waiting lists and many patients having, in effect, no access to hospital or primary care. This presents doctors with a real moral dilemma. Is it better to apply the highest standards, and give adequate time for communication to a few patients, knowing that to do so will reduce dramatically the number of patients that can be dealt with, even if this leads to lengthening waiting times and denial of access for other patients? Or should one compromise and, on the principles of utilitarianism, seek the greatest good for the greatest number? This means cutting corners, packing the patients in, and getting the job done, so that most patients can be dealt with in a reasonable time, though not necessarily in the manner that modern consumerism demands—let alone what the GMC would wish. Is it to be a 'Rolls-Royce' service for the few, or a rushed and compromised service for the many? It is a real dilemma, and most doctors opt for the latter approach (and were they in any doubt, their hospital mangers would clarify the issue for them).

In short, most doctors prefer to give as many patients as possible access to health care, if only to perform triage and to identify urgent cases at an early stage. So deep down every doctor knows that to follow *all* the GMC's advice on standards and communication and training is incompatible with *real* medical practice in the hurly burly of the NHS. Perhaps the *quid pro quo* for the doctor accepting revalidation might be a better understanding by the GMC that most of life is a compromise and nowhere more so than when trying to reconcile the impossible demands of modern medicine with the high standards that doctors wish to practise. The GMC must be equally willing, when investigating under-performance, to point the finger at inadequate funding, poor facilities and excessive workload as it is to identify deficiencies in individual doctors.

An Independent Medical Inspectorate
A Proposal to Promote Patient Benefit By Encouraging Medical Openness and the Clinical Accountability of Medical Staff in the UK

William G. Pickering

This chapter describes the reasons and need for an independent medical inspectorate, and how it could be instituted within the NHS and the private sector. Such a body would be impartial and informed, and it would concern itself primarily with clinical matters. Thus, waiting lists, appointment delays, numbers of prescriptions or operations, and other heterogeneous quantitative matters, would *not* be within its remit. Neither, in the first instance at least, would it concern itself with tactlessness, impoliteness or insensitivity—which too are very important matters (sometimes more important than pure clinical issues).[1] Rather, its prime function would be to concentrate on the identification of the qualitative issue of sub-standard clinical practice and, by feeding back information of such findings to doctors, it would start to make the medical profession accountable for its clinical actions. Accountability in other walks of life, exacted by an outside statutory body, is thought unambiguously to raise standards of quality within the examined profession. There is every reason to believe that this would also apply to medical practice. Considering what is at stake (the well-being of patients), some will think it surprising that the medical profession has to date, except via civil litigation, avoided (or escaped) being externally accountable for its clinical actions. This is particularly evident in general practice, where clinical accountability is virtually non-existent: but it is also minimal in parts of hospital practice and in private practice.

There are episodic medical disasters which make it to the popular press and prompt attention. Certain substandard medical screening tests, occurring in very large numbers, provide one recent example. Another was 'the Bristol case' debacle. Here, 29 children met their deaths. It might have been thought that one unusual death would have prompted an investigation, or certainly that two would have. In the event, ten did not: even 20 did not. And yet, dead children are easily counted. This was not a subtle or obscure matter to record. The point is that, if, to focus attention and attract recognition, disasters have to occur in these large numbers in one place, what chance is there to uncover single episodes of substandard medicine in general practice and hospitals throughout the country on a daily basis? The answer is more or less no chance—as patients well know. All processions of medical disasters, however, begin with a single disaster.

As if to underline this apparent necessity of a sequence of disasters before action is taken, there has been the recent Shipman case. One important reason that the chilling events in Hyde began, and then continued for so long, was because their perpetrator knew that in the NHS, and in general practice in particular, doctors can do more or less what they like. They call it 'clinical freedom' and cherish it. No one (except the law) can meaningfully challenge their actions, and then only if they are found out. As usual, it was left to patients and the press to blow the whistle. Had it been left to the self-regulatory bodies—the GMC, royal colleges or local medical personnel, the disaster could well have been continuing still. We might ask those medico-politicians who have commented that this was a 'one-off' case: as there is no effective mechanism to uncover even such terrible irregularities as this, how would anyone know this is a one-off? 'Self-regulation' of doctors is, self-evidently, equivalent to no regulation. The unhindered sequence of Shipman's exploits begs, amongst others, the recurring and uncomfortable question pertaining to day-to-day clinical medicine. If that extreme of behaviour could not be stopped until the victim numbers reached double figures, what chance is there to uncover single instances of poor clinical medicine and stop them recurring?

At the outset, it should be made clear that the clinical matters to which an inspectorate would apply itself would be ones very basic and rudimentary to medical practice. The standard of practice expected would be that which any 'reasonably competent' doctor (as the law puts it) could be expected to provide. Two absolute priorities would be, firstly, the unnecessarily late diagnosis of treatable disease; and secondly, the improper supervision of ongoing medical treatment. On the other hand, rarer or 'small print' diagnosis would be of interest only if the doctor had strayed from basic medical rules in the search for a diagnosis. For example, it may be shown that a doctor had ignored some red cells (blood) in a urine test of a male patient, who a year later was found to have a tumour within the urinary tract. The issue would not be that the doctor had missed until late an uncommon but perhaps lethal condition, but that he or she had ignored a year ago a very fundamental and basic abnormality in a urine test (ordered by the doctor), which, if noticed and followed up, might have led to earlier referral and diagnosis. This would very probably have been to the patient's advantage. To continue with this example: medical students are taught not to ignore such things as blood in the urine. If they do so in their final exams they may fail them because the reason *for* tests is precisely to act on any such abnormality. This is very basic medicine. To repeat, an inspectorate would not concern itself with the slow recognition of obscure presentations of either common or uncommon diseases. Its domain would be the elementary ground rules of medicine. It is well known that in the police force it is the following of basic and routine procedures, rather than inspiration, which usually solves simple and difficult cases alike: but omission or neglect of this rudimentary method can lead to delay or worse. This analogy is applicable to medical practice.

Accountability Of Doctors And Patients

Whilst it is true that nobody is perfect, not least members of the medical profession, a person attending for a professional medical opinion is entitled to 'reasonable competence' from the doctor. By and large this usually happens. Sometimes patients receive from their doctor exceptional diagnostic and management expertise. Indeed, the quality of NHS medicine varies from excellent to poor. It is very educative to peruse cases where all the records are available, such as those which come to medical litigation. Here, in black and white, is seen a spectrum of circumstances ranging from rank medical negligence to vexatious patient litigiousness. The latter often occurs where the doctor(s) have practised exemplary medicine, only to end up being sued. Which brings us to another useful, albeit secondary, function of a medical inspectorate. It would not only make doctors accountable: it would have the capacity to make patients accountable too. The advantages of this for doctors, in the context of being victims of groundless but nonetheless unsettling clinical complaints, are obvious. This even-handedness might make their own clinical accountability a less bitter pill to swallow.

Moreover, quite separately from litigation, some patients are known to abuse the medical services.[2] An inspectorate would, as with poor clinical practice by doctors, not let this pass without, at the very least, remark. As has been noted, when patients abuse their rights to medical care they do so much to the detriment of other patients and the service providers.[3] In its way this is every bit as important a matter as errant doctors, and they both need urgent attention.[4]

The Longstanding Impediments To Medical Glasnost

The medical profession feels, naturally, that to do its job it must be allowed to take a full history from patients and, when necessary, perform a full examination of them. It is expected of the users of health services that, for their health's sake, they will noiselessly submit to these things. It is perhaps an irony, then, that the medical profession is so reluctant to occasionally (for *its* health's sake) be properly examined itself. But, as is well known, it delights in autonomy and 'self-regulation'. Some doctors may, with undisguised irritation, rebut this statement of fact. They might cite the multiplicity of audits to which they are now subject: numbers of patients seen, numbers of prescriptions issued, etc. However, if one measures, say, the number of prescriptions issued and dispensed (in itself a not unimportant matter), one still has not the slightest clue as to what happens to the patients who swallow the medicines actually given. Did they benefit from their medicines or not? We have no idea.[5] Measuring numbers, then, tells little or nothing about quality of care. A medical inspector-ate would be, uniquely, an instrument of qualitative audit, and one in touch with daily medical practice. To use an analogy, traffic police, rather than counting erring drivers, stop them singly and remark upon it. Not only is the driver's mind concentrated but that of others too. Just the presence of one police car alters the behaviour of hundreds of drivers. There is an immediacy about an inspectorate, whose function would be first to identify those who drive through clinical red lights (irrespective of their rank or status)—and then promptly to bring it to their attention. Nothing in the health services has ever done this, which is why bad practice continues to coexist with all the good practice.

In the same vein, sundry new propositions are currently 'doing the rounds, invented (by doctors or politicians) to deal in part with the issue of quality, or perhaps designed in part to placate critics. Peer assessment, reaccreditation of doctors, governance, institutes for clinical excellence, commissions for health improvement are some of the galaxy of suggestions.[6] There may be first class reasons for their eventual implementation; but, lest there be any misunderstanding, they are *not* the same as impartial, informed accountability for daily clinical practice. They are not devoted to uncovering single, sporadic medical errors (which is how most occur), they are not impartial, and there is every indication that rather than being independent, they are, albeit under different names, self-regulation redesigned. The archi-tects or implementers of any new initiative pertaining to clinical 'quality' must ask themselves the following questions. Has it a chance of promptly picking up any single instances of sub-optimal clinical practice, countrywide, on a daily basis? Could it possibly pick up the case depicted above (p. 48), or the first or second of a series of surgical blunders? There is another question. Could such bodies, whatever their alleged merits, actually risk obscuring the identification of poor practice by giving the noisy impression they are doing something about it?

There is a longstanding view amongst doctors that they should be unquestioningly permitted 'clinical freedom'. This term has somehow acquired the status of a divine medical right, and anything which compromises its implicit message has been resisted at all costs. That message is medical autonomy, which is to say the facility, when one is a doctor, to do what one wants. Depending on the ability, the intellect, the sensibility and the energy of its exponents, the best and the worst of medical practice have resulted. 'Clinical freedom' is the antithesis of medical openness and the very opposite of medical *glasnost*. The mentality which devised the term and doggedly clings to it, and which haughtily uses it to deny access of others to the medical *modus operandi*, is the mentality which prevents true and consistent quality from percolating throughout health services. Yet practice which takes account of whether there was or was not patient benefit ensuing from medical intervention, and practice which has clearly obeyed rudimentary medical rules, has nothing to fear, one would imagine, from, on occasion, opening its doors and records to such a body as an inspectorate, especially as the beneficiaries will be users of the health services. 'Clinical freedom' can only be retained if the results of 'clinical freedom' are acceptable. It requires periodic examination of its results if it is to continue. Basic medical error, unnecessarily late diagnosis, improper supervision of medical treatment etc., cannot continue to pass without remark, record or question. As aggrieved patients will testify, it is as though such regrettable outcomes have been enacted by some omniscient medical being, with whom such sub-optimal results are mysteriously unrelated and which, anyway, were unavoidable. Quite often, nothing could be further from the truth.

Complaints, Impartiality, And The Inspectorate

There is much clamour at the present time to produce an effective system for dealing with patient complaints, both in the hospital and general practice spheres. It is clearly important to deal with them properly and to resolve them to the satisfaction of the patient (and medical staff), if at all possible. Their proper management is felt by some to be the key to medical quality. If complaints are properly addressed, it is assumed, then quality in the NHS will improve. Complaints are thought by some to be one real route to exact accountability upon a profession who hitherto has avoided it. Unfortunately, as things stand, they are not. It is possible for new 'local resolution' procedures to be carried out without the doctor involved ever knowing anything of the complaint. Also, these procedures are not necessarily patient-friendly. Is it reasonable to ask a patient (or their relative) who has been the victim of indifferent clinical practice to first take their grievance to the very practice or hospital which perpetrated it? Above all, impartiality, i.e. freedom from the local medical brotherhood, is not evident in current procedures. Also, an informed opinion about a clinical matter just cannot be provided by lay people (practice mangers, complaints managers, conveners, independent lay people).

The two essential requirements for decent handling of complaints are 1) an impartial opinion and 2) an informed opinion and explanation. Both are missing in the current 'new' complaints procedures. Even assuming they may possibly work for non-clinical matters (cold food, long appointment waiting times, impolite staff), for the serious matter of alleged clinical mismanagement there is every chance they will be as unsuccessful (more so possibly) as previous systems. In some ways the new and current state of affairs, partial, ill-informed and adversarial as it is, seems designed to deter or even stop people complaining. Unsurprisingly, anecdotal reports in the early days of these new NHS complaints procedures already suggest less use of them, particularly of the 'local resolution' procedures. It is at this very crucial first point of complaint that an inspectorate would insist upon information. A copy of all these complaints would be passed to the inspectorate, and the patients would know of this. The copy would have on it the name of the person who was dealing with it. Patients would know that an impartial, informed body had record of, and could, if indicated, investigate complaints, thus pressing 'local resolution' personnel to deal scrupulously with things at the outset. It would also urge certain patients to be less fanciful and more accurate with the facts of their complaints.

The Categorisation Of Complaints Into Clinical And Non-Clinical

The inspectorate would also insist that 'local resolution' staff (doctors obviously should be involved here) immediately ascribe complaints arriving at their door or hospital as 'clinical' or 'non-clinical'. Note that the question of whether a complaint has within it a clinical element is not always easily or accurately disentangled by a lay person. If there is doubt, then they must be labelled 'clinical'. This is to insist that a habitual mentality of clinical accountability take firm root in practices and hospitals. Besides a copy of the complaint, 'local resolution' staff would also send a copy of the written reply sent to the patient to the inspectorate (with its contained explanation and, if necessary, its apology). The complainant would be informed of this too. Whether there has been medical error or fault, or excellent medical attention and the patient has misread what has taken place (this is not uncommon), there would at least be an official record. And if there appeared to be a discrepancy between the complaint and the reply/explanation, then the inspectorate would be at liberty to investigate the matter further, including full scrutiny of the medical records. Complaints can be one very useful guide to the efficacy or otherwise of medical intervention and to the quality thereof. Private clinical practice and private hospitals would, like the NHS, also be obliged to pass a copy of received complaints, and response, to the inspectorate. Similarly, availability of access to their records would be necessary.

Practices, health authorities and trusts would be required to publish an annual report on complaints received (in a standard and analysable form specified by the inspectorate), including whether they were deemed clinical or non-clinical and why, and what action was taken. It should be remembered that it is intended that less than competent clinical practice should, in so far as possible, not any longer be able to pass without remark or record.

The inspectorate would aim to dovetail into current or new systems. That is, no major upheaval in current personnel is envisaged. There is however something of an upheaval in the mentality envisaged.

Other Related Extant Bodies, Including The Dental Reference Officer.

The GMC's function is, as their slogan puts it, to 'protect patients and guide doctors'. In line with fashion, it has now added 'professional performance procedures'[7] to its current 'doctors' conduct and health procedures', which are 'to investigate cases where there is evidence that a doctor's general performance is seriously deficient'. (Why has this only happened now and not decades ago? To comply with fashion and avoid public and political criticism or obloquy, one presumes). These new 'procedures' talk of identifying a 'general pattern' of poor performance, and of 'repeated and persistent failure'. These rather bureaucratic and constraining terms appear to some people an obstacle to its fluid and regular use for identification of sub-standard medicine. There are added problems. Most people do not know of the GMC's existence, let alone its phone number. Thus most of its received queries and complaints arise from hospital trusts (which naturally are aware of it), whilst allegations of bad general practice from less well-informed patients are few. Exactly who should contact the GMC with a problem and who should go through NHS complaint procedures is unclear, and this confusion naturally acts as a deterrent to patients. It would be helpful to all if the GMC could spell out its precise niche with regard to clinical accountability. No matter how many lay persons it employs in its 'performance procedures', the GMC, the very organisation which registers doctors, is unlikely ever to persuade patients that it is impartial. Furthermore, it is dauntingly immured in central London: the assessment of day-to-day clinical quality (or the contrary) in the NHS throughout the country is therefore quite beyond it. An inspectorate, by contrast, would be broadly based, eventually with a presence in each region throughout the country. Also, it would not constrain itself with terms like 'pattern' or 'repeated and persistent' failure of doctors' actions, but would look open-mindedly at any allegation of clinical ineptitude which it received. There is a distinct impression that the GMC is a little 'picky' when it comes to exactly which clinical complaints it will permit itself to deal with. On its own, the remote and lumbering GMC is never, if past form and current plans are any guide, going to be sufficiently adept, nimble and promptly effective at identifying poor clinical practice as is an inspectorate. If there were to be some link up between an inspectorate (the findings thereof) and the GMC, then this latter body would have to prepare and equip itself for an undreamed-of increase in workload, and change in mentality.

In passing, it is quite wrong to split doctors, as the GMC proposes for example, into good performers and bad performers in the belief that poor practice can be somehow spotted from a distance—via, say, the layout of the surgery or the state of the medical records or periodic re-examination. It usually cannot. Sub-optimal clinical practice can emerge from highly qualified, 'well-thought-of' sources. Furthermore, those who feel that more education (albeit laudable in itself) is the answer to poor medicine must understand it does not obviate the need for clinical accountability. Amongst the recent high-profile cases dealt with by the GMC, there has been no shortage of qualifications or college status amongst the alleged errant doctors. Would driving a well kept car, or re-passing the driving test every few years, obviate the need for traffic police? It would not. The only way to identify and pick up sporadic clinical errors made by doctors is to specifically look for them, all the time, irrespective of the age or rank of the doctor. There is no alternative. The simplicity of this seems, to bemused patients, to have been an impediment to its implementation.

In the Bristol case, the GMC availed themselves to assess the culprits. However, it was, alas, left to the parents and the media to uncover the debacle. If it had been left to the GMC, the grim events at Bristol would have been continuing still. So far as the identification throughout the country of substandard clinical practice is concerned, the GMC is irrelevant.

The remit of the health service ombudsman has recently been extended to clinical issues. It does not take all complaints. It is not an alternative to NHS procedures. It is essential to have gone through NHS procedures before prevailing upon the ombudsman, who is only used if there is a *prima facie* case that the NHS system of resolution has failed the patient. Although the ombudsman is a constitutional safeguard for citizens, although it is in part a monitor of indifferent clinical practice, and although it is independent of the NHS, it is not accessible for most clinical complaints (dealing with only 338 grievances in 1995-96, less than a fifth of which were upheld[8]). It is therefore ineffective as a potent tool to exact clinical accountability and, as far as maintaining clinical standards is concerned, irrelevant. Notwithstanding, it is worth pointing out that (like an inspectorate) it *is* impartial and informed—and it is interesting that the government thinks that such a body, however small and, relatively speaking, inconsequential to most complainants, is nonetheless an essential safeguard for patients and quality. Tokenism perhaps, but it is a sort of inspectorate.

Dental reference officers (DROs), who work for the governmental department known as the Dental Practice Board (DPB),[9] are public servants who are independent clinicians (i.e. qualified dentists) giving independent advice. Although their remit is quite extensive (including looking at financial issues) they are, in part, an independent quality inspectorate, carrying out quality monitoring of dentistry. Part of the NHS contract of dentists insists that they will be subject to this monitoring. The health authority has the power, if necessary, to fine errant dentists. Interestingly, the government has decided to *increase* the number of DROs, such is their value. There is one current problem, in that private dental practice (as opposed to NHS practice) is not subject to their scrutiny: certain information suggests this situation may soon be rectified. Clearly there are very important parallels between DROs and a medical inspectorate. They do not have exactly the same brief; the medical version would have a narrower one, concentrating mostly on clinical matters. However, clinical accountability exacted by an outside (non-NHS) organisation is not a new idea. It is just that it has been restricted to dentistry: clinical medicine remains, by contrast, inexplicably exempt. If it is right to make dentists accountable to an impartial inspectorate, it is naturally right to extend this to doctors.

Further Reasons Why Poor Clinical Practice Passes Without Remark

It has to be remembered that a great number of justifiably aggrieved patients, for various reasons—embarrassment, fear of meeting the medical brotherhood's stonewall, or of being ejected from a doctor's list, for example—never complain. As a consequence, the occurrence or incidence of much poor medical practice is never divulged to anyone but close relatives and friends. Officially it does not exist. So, befuddlement on anti-depressants, addiction to tranquillisers, bleeding from anti-inflammatory drugs, urinary tract infections missed in children, unreferred breast lumps, unnoticed abnormal laboratory test results, unnecessarily late diagnoses of treatable disease, etc., pass weekly without even official remark, let alone action, comment or intervention. Small wonder they continue. It is as though our current medical system, in tandem with the understandable human trait extant in some patients not 'to cause a stir', unite to obscure medical errors and mismanagements, rather than to highlight and acknowledge them, which would help to deter and minimise their occurrence.

On a similar theme, great care should be taken in the interpretation of numbers of civil medical litigation cases brought. In order to be in receipt of legal aid (i.e. legal expenses paid) one has to have few or no financial resources. So, those people reasonably well-off but not rich (a sizeable proportion of the population) will not resort to litigation for alleged medical negligence. This is not because they may not have a notable case, but because they cannot afford it. When these people do not (for various reasons) use the complaints system and then cannot use the legal system because of cost, their case too (be it with or without foundation) is unrecorded.

Methods Other Than Complaints Of Identifying Poor Clinical Practice

Very few medical students, sitting alongside consultants in hospital out-patients, have not noticed that occasional GP referral letters, when read in conjunction with the patient's current history and condition, clearly denote that the GP is late in his or her referral, or has been mismanaging things. For example, a person with rectal bleeding for a year has been diagnosed by the GP during that year as having haemorrhoids, only to eventually develop pain and weight loss and to be only then referred. A basic history and examination (i.e. nothing sophisticated, expensive or subtle) at the outset (a year ago), or a definitive instruction to the patient to come back to the GP for review in, say, a month's time, may well have defined that the patient's symptoms were by no means certainly those of haemorrhoids (for which dietary advice and a cream were advised) but indicated more serious and sinister problems. It is a source of great surprise to most students and junior doctors that a definitive message is not sent by the consultant in the letter to the GP that they should endeavour not to make this mistake again. The young doctor, however, soon learns that one can do anything in medicine except that which may be construed as criticism of a professional colleague's clinical practice. The referral letter from GP to hospital which, together with the patient's condition, define poor practice (as well as excellent practice sometimes) must not be diplomatically ignored by hospital consultants any longer. They are a potent source of qualitative information about clinical practice and, when necessary, they must (as a condition of service) be brought to the notice of an inspectorate. Similarly, information after hospital referral or treatment must be passed on, where applicable, by GPs. It is not so much a question of 'whistle blowing', it is a question of forcing doctors to review their *modus operandi* in the interests of patient benefit. If there are any beneficiaries resulting from the traditional and hitherto unbreachable wall of medical silence, then the users of the health services are not amongst them.

Some hospital researchers are now occasionally actually publishing work spelling out that long delays occur in the diagnosis of patients with some potentially treatable cancers.[10] This is only documenting what every doctor, nurse and medical student has always known. The unnecessarily late diagnosis of various treatable diseases, including cancer, has been happening for decades on quite a large scale. Most pass officially without remark, and still we await the definitive remedy for stopping it repeatedly occurring. An inspectorate would focus very strongly on this lamentable situation. Of course, there are many diseases other than cancer which are improved by earlier rather than later diagnosis. To repeat, this does not automatically imply that more money need be spent on more referrals or on sophisticated investigations. Routine medical histories and examinations, and reasonably competent interpretation thereof, are the issue. This is not a matter of obsessively and unrealistically preaching the unachievable merit of perfection. It is simply one of the reinforcement of those basic principles and methods which were, and still are, the major part of medical training.

Disease Caused By Medical Intervention

Iatrogenesis is the official name for disease caused by medicine and doctors. It is not a deeply researched topic. Few medical personnel see any personal gain or career enhancement in looking at diseases caused by the medical profession; but it is an important topic. It is estimated that over five per cent of hospital admissions are caused by medical treatments.[11] It might appear to be priority information that certain actions in medicine and surgery have caused disease requiring admission, and that such events, such hospital admissions, such morbidity and mortality, should be assiduously categorised and recorded as such. But they are not. There are also very substantial undisclosed numbers of doctor-caused diseases evident in general practice which never reach hospital. Nearly all are publicly unrecorded. Thousands of people over at least two decades were subjected relentlessly (by prescribing and repeat prescribing) to the addictive properties of long-term benzodiazepine 'tranquillisers', before their ill-effects were at last noticed and prescribing began to diminish. That is a long time for bad practice to continue unaltered. It demonstrates that those systems in operation for reporting, say, adverse drug reactions[12] are singularly ineffective. It is rare for more than ten per cent of serious reactions to be reported; and in general reporting is rarely better than two to four per cent.[13] It also begs the very important question: if poor practice on a scale of thousands of cases cannot be publicly uncovered for decades, what are the chances, as things stand, of uncovering poor practice on the smaller, per-doctor-per-person scale?

The key questions that are not habitually and regularly asked by doctors are:

1)   did the patient benefit from medical intervention?

2)   did they not?

3)   were they made worse?

Would long-term benzodiazepines have been so recklessly prescribed if these questions had been asked? The evidence of addiction and their uselessness at solving the patient's original problem was always there for every prescribing doctor to see. Doctors either closed their eyes or they ignored the evidence of their own observations. One wonders what current therapies will soon be shown to have been a dangerous fashion? The side-effects of NSAI drugs, for example, are often more evident than their efficacy.[14] An inspectorate could not overnight put into operation all the key initiatives necessary to answer the above three questions every time a doctor sees a patient, particularly as such daily objectivity has been so steadfastly avoided for so long. But it is the responsibility of each practising doctor to be habitually objective about what they are doing. The sneering academic accusations that clinical observations are invalid (compared to big trials) because they are merely 'anecdotal' is precisely the mentality which discourages initiative amongst doctors and does nothing to improve clinical quality.[15]

As its main role is clinical accountability, an inspectorate would be in a good position to start to raise the profile of the matter of both patient benefit and iatrogenesis to everyday matters. It has been said that 'with iatrogenic illness, as with many other diseases, prevention is the best course of action'.[16] But, alas, it seems currently that the outcome of medical intervention is seen by many doctors to be of less importance than its actuation.[17] Complaints with regard to drugs, and hospital admissions caused by medicines or medical intervention, should be documented as such, and the inspectorate informed. Unfortunately there is particularly poor reporting of serious drug reactions by all hospital doctors, despite the fact that these events are most likely to present in hospital.[18] This inactivity, this cover-up, has to stop. Conventional rules for reporting adverse drug events must, of course, continue, but an inspectorate may well be able to provide the Committee on Safety of Medicines with important further information.

Patient Satisfaction

The contemporary public and political obsession with patient satisfaction, which, for better or worse, has spilled into the medical profession, is very relevant to any discussion about clinical accountability and how to exact it. Long before patient satisfaction became enshrined in daily lay edicts, doctors usually intuitively aimed to achieve this very thing, and historically probably always have done. But now the slogan has become for some groups a *sine qua non* for health service 'quality'. If the patient is dissatisfied then the profession, some think, has failed them. This is a very serious mistake.[19] It can mean that doctors become puppets of their patients who, as often as not, hold mistaken medical perceptions of what they need. A man with headaches might feel he needs a skull X-ray or hospital referral and scan. His GP, after a careful history and examination, may feel he needs neither after diagnosing and painstakingly explaining to the patient that his problems are benign and self-limiting. The man may be dissatisfied. He may be referred because the GP is brow-beaten. The consultant may agree that the problem is benign but orders a scan—for a quiet life: the scan, as expected is normal. All this happens regularly. Doctors can be forced into inessential tests, medications, referrals, investigations and operations. The waste and expense are obvious. Also, the patient can be subjected to harm from such tests and medications. The salient point here is that patient satisfaction is not by any means always equivalent to sound medical practice. Patient dissatisfaction can result from excellent medical practice. It is an inconvenient fact that fulsome medical explanation often does not persuade some patients of the inapplicability of some of their fanciful medical notions. When complaints ensue (e.g. 'the doctor refused me an X-ray', 'refused to refer me' etc.), an inspectorate's support may be needed to unravel some of these matters. It is essential that doctors are allowed to treat on medical grounds alone. Note also that one of the beneficiaries here, as it happens, will be health services' finances.

Lessons From The Law

Much can be learnt from medico-legal cases which is germane to clinical accountability and the inception of an inspectorate.

a) It is deemed mandatory by solicitors to obtain copies of *all* the medical records. This is because it is felt (correctly) that no case of alleged clinical negligence can be decently addressed without them. An inspectorate must, when the occasion demands, at least have access to them too. (Do current clinical complaints at the NHS gate routinely have all their clinical records examined? They do not.)

b) Solicitors themselves do not prepare the medical report, though of course they read the records and the client statement. The preparation of a definitive medical report (upon which rest legal decisions about whether to proceed with the case or not) is done by a medical person. An impartial one is sought—though not always found. Even the law sometimes has difficulty in finding an impartial doctor to provide a report, so ingrained is the tendency to medical defensiveness. What chance, then, have NHS in-house complaint systems of impartially attending to allegations of clinical ineptitude?

c) The reason that solicitors themselves could not prepare these reports is, of course, because they have no working knowledge of medicine. Yet current NHS complaints processes are governed by lay-persons—presumably to assure everyone there will be fair and unbiased play—even when purely clinical matters are under review. It is not that lay people are unimportant, it is just that they are medically uninformed. It is a very grave error to assume that because lay people are involved then the matters are therefore properly examined, and the method is irreproachable. An inspectorate may not obviate the need for some involvement of lay persons but, by contrast, it is not uninformed, whilst it still has the impartiality of a lay person. It is less likely to ignore or overlook the clinical matters which need urgent attention. It is more likely to be able quickly to sift and prioritise complaints that it proposes to examine. Also, it can interpret records without difficulty. It must also be able to work harmoniously with those lay people currently involved in these matters.

It is implied by some people that the actual recognition of poor medical practice is difficult. 'There are so many things to consider', 'medicine is not all black and white, you know' and similar exculpatory remarks have been heard by many complainants. In truth, as anyone who has examined medico-legal cases will know (and where all the medical records were available), the decision as to whether or not there has been less than 'reasonably competent' practice is seldom difficult. It is usually easy (the medical employees of medical defence organisations, for example, do it day in and day out). It is important to realise this, for an inspectorate would be able to be pretty decisive one way or the other. And, depending upon its findings, it would be able to inform the doctor appropriately, in language which is clear and intelligible.

It is often said by persons who feel aggrieved by actual or perceived medical mismanagement that they simply want:

1) an explanation of what happened

2) an apology

3) reassurance that it will not happen to someone else.[20]

In medico-legal cases there is (or should be) a jargon-free report of events: of what happened and what didn't happen. Sometimes the client remarks that this is the first time they have been told exactly what happened. Whether or not there has been medical negligence, it is usually an immense relief for them to understand the train of events. If provision of an explanation from the in-house procedures is deemed by the inspectorate to be inadequate (having received a copy), then the inspectorate could, when necessary, insist on a fuller report being given to the complainant. Every encouragement would be given to those staffing the existing procedures to produce the goods. If there has been less than reasonable medical competence shown, the offending doctor can (when prompted by the inspectorate) provide the apology. If nothing else is achieved, then the patient will know that the matter has not been swept under the carpet. But moreover, the conspicuous identification of events, and notification thereof to the parties involved, is likely to provide the aggrieved patient with evidence that this is (now) much less likely to happen to someone else. If, on the other hand, it is shown that the doctor's management of things was impeccable, and that the patient has misrepresented or misinterpreted events, then this information also is made clear to all—so deterring any time-wasting and frivolous complaints.

Summary

- An independent medical inspectorate, whilst not a panacea for all the ills of the health services, would appraise and ventilate certain clinical events. When necessary it would require a doctor to account for an episode, or episodes, of their clinical practice. This procedure is inseparably connected to what happens to patients after medical intervention.

- Its implementation, by engendering a healthy atmosphere of openness, would be likely to raise clinical standards, raise morale in medical staff and patients, and increase patient confidence in medical competence.

- Its primary aim would be to identify poor clinical practice which currently passes without even remark, let alone official recognition: and to inform those involved of its findings. Clinical accountability of medical personnel would begin to become a reality.

- The corollary to its work, it is hoped, would be to help prevent future (and similar) errors.

- To some extent, patients too would become accountable.

- It would exist in addition to the current complaints systems, complementing them and making them more effective in improving clinical practice.

- It would also exist in addition to all the other lesser known avenues available (actual or theoretical ones) to patients, such as the GMC and the health services ombudsman.

- It would exist *alongside* any new 'initiatives' such as those currently envisaged.[21] Indeed, all such bodies should be intimately associated with the findings of an inspectorate.

- It would concentrate upon the departure from rudimentary clinical method.

- It would not specifically concern itself with 'small print' medical minutiae.

- It would raise the profile and importance of 'patient benefit' from medical intervention.

- It would raise the profile of iatrogenesis and its prevention.

- It would aim to deter treatment by rote (as with some medications and operations) for which benefit is not always evident.

- It would not be a 'second opinion' for patients or for doctors.

- It would require to be informed of poor clinical practice by both hospital doctors (when they see it) and general practitioners (when they see it). Suppression of such information has to date not benefited patients. A culture of openness (not reproach) would be nurtured in the interests of quality. Private medicine would, similarly, be open to scrutiny.

- Although complaints would not be the only source of information for an inspectorate, it would require to see copies of all complaints *and* their responses. The authorities (NHS and private) would label them 'clinical' or 'non-clinical', but, in the first instance at least, all would have to be seen by the inspectorate.

- It could not, for the time being anyway, look at the very important matters of politeness and tact. To repeat, its primary aim would be identification of poor clinical method.

- It is to be hoped that if there are any persons unenthusiastic about accountability they will desist from the customary grumbles of this being 'just another layer of bureaucracy'. A medical inspectorate would be possessed of qualities which are not invariably associated with bureaucracies or self-regulatory bodies, such as impartiality, initiative, sensibility, purpose, promptitude and effectiveness. It would also be inexpensive.

- It could not look at financial issues. However, if treatment by rote is deterred, and patient benefit (rather than patient satisfaction) is held at the forefront, then it is highly likely some savings would be made, perhaps substantial ones. Also, when standards improve (by the mere presence of an inspectorate) it is likely that litigation and its extravagant cost to health services would diminish.

- The medical inspector would be medically qualified. He or she, whilst working in a trust and/or health authority, would not be paid by the NHS but centrally. Some evident track-record of interest, insight and experience of medical disputes/complaints/qualitative assessment of medical practice/sovereign role of patient benefit, would be necessary.

- A pilot scheme for an inspectorate, in a district or region, with all the relevant personnel being properly informed (and their co-operation sought) is urgently recommended. Eventually a nation-wide network of 50 to 60 inspectors is envisaged.

- It may be expected that in time, perhaps a very short time, as a different mentality takes root—an objective and open one—the intervention of an inspectorate would be minimal.

Notes

David Gladstone

1   Kelleher, D., Gabe, J. and Williams, G., 'Understanding medical dominance in the modern world', in Gabe, J. *et al.* (eds.), *Challenging Medicine*, London: Routledge, 1994, p .xiii.

2   The Rt. Hon. Alan Milburn, Secretary of State for Health, Statement in House of Commons, 1 February 2000. Cited in *The Times*, 2 February 2000, p. 1.

3   Perkin, H., *The Rise of Professional Society: England Since 1880*, London: Routledge, 1989, pp. 472-73.

4   For further discussion see Gladstone, D., 'Doctor and patient, state and market', in Phillips, C.I. (ed.), *Logic in Medicine* (2nd edition), London: B.M.J. Publishing Group, 1995, pp. 193-210; and Gladstone, D. and Goldsmith, M., 'Health care reform in the UK: working for patients?', in Seedhouse, D. (ed.), *Reforming Health Care*, Chichester: John Wiley and Sons, 1995, pp. 71-84.

5   Porter, R., *Disease, Medicine and Society in England 1550-1860*, London: Macmillan, 1987, p. 52.

6   Stewart, J., 'Accountability and empowerment in welfare services', in Gladstone, D. (ed.), *British Social Welfare: Past, Present and Future*, London: UCL Press, 1995, p. 289.

7   Hart, N., *The Sociology of Health and Medicine*, Ormskirk: Causeway Press, 1985, p. 101.

8   Allsop, J., 'Two sides to every story: complainants' and doctors' perspectives in disputes about medical care in a general practice setting', *Law and Policy*, Vol. 16, No. 2, 1994.

Brian Salter

1   Allsop, J. and Mulcahy, L., *Regulating Medical Work: Formal and Informal Controls*, Buckingham: Open University Press, 1996.

2   Stacey, M., 'The GMC and professional accountability', *Public Policy and Administration*, Vol. 4, No. 1, 1989, p. 15.

3   Hafferty, F.W. and McKinlay, J.B., *The Changing Medical Profession: An International Perspective*, Oxford: Oxford University Press, 1993; Moran, M. and Wood, B., *States, Regulation and the Medical Profession*, Buckingham: Open University Press, 1993.

4   Stacey, M., *Regulating British Medicine: The General Medical Council*, London: John Wiley, 1992, ch. 3.

5   Merrison Committee (Chair: Sir Alec Merrison), *Report of the Committee of Inquiry into the Regulation of the Medical Profession*, Cmnd. 6018, London: HMSO, 1975, p. 3.

6 Allsop and Mulcahy, *Regulating Medical Work*, 1996, chs. 4 and 5.

7 British Medical Association, Academy of Medical Royal Colleges, Joint Consultants Committee, *Making Self-regulation Work at the Local Level*, London: BMA, 1998.

8 Stacey, *Regulating British Medicine*,1992, p. 219.

9 Haug, M., 'Deprofessionalisation: an alternative hypothesis for the future', *Sociological Review Monograph*, Vol. 20, 1973, pp. 195-211; Haug, M., 'A re-examination of the hypothesis of deprofessionalisation', *The Millbank Quarterly,* Vol. 66 (suppl. 2), 1988, pp. 48-56; Starr, P. *The Social Transformation of American Medicine*, New York: Basic Books, 1982.

10 Ernst, E., 'The rise and fall of complementary medicine', *Journal of the Royal Society of Medicine*, Vol. 91, No. 5, 1998, pp. 235-36; Fisher, P. and Ward, A., 'Complementary medicine in Europe', *British Medical Journal*, Vol. 309, 1994, pp. 107-11.

11 Blume, S., *Insight and Industry: on the Dynamics of Technological Change in Medicine,* Cambridge, Mass: MIT Press, 1992; Wickham, I., 'An introduction to minimally invasive surgery', *Health Policy*, Vol. 23, 1993, pp. 7-15.

12 Allsop and Mulcahy, *Regulating Medical Work*, 1996, chs. 7 and 9; Moran, M. 'Explaining change in the NHS: corporatism, closure and democratic capitalism', *Public Policy and Administration*, Vol. 10, No. 2, 1995, p. 30.

13 'The dark side of medicine', *British Medical Journal*, Vol. 316, 1998, p. 1733.

14 Klein, R., 'Competence, professional self-regulation, and the public interest' *British Medical Journal,* Vol. 316, 1998, p. 1740.

15 Smith, R., 'The future of the GMC: an interview with Donald Irvine, the new president', *British Medical Journal*, Vol. 310, 1995, p. 1516.

16 Klein, 'Competence, professional self-regulation, and the public interest', 1998, p. 1742.

17 MacPherson, G., '1948: a turbulent gestation for the NHS', *British Medical Journal*, Vol. 316, 1998, p. 6.

18 Klein, R., *The Politics of the NHS*, London: Longman, 1989, p. 82.

19 Moran, 'Explaining change in the NHS: corporatism, closure and democratic capitalism', 1995, p. 31.

20 Salter, B., *The Politics of Change in the Health Service,* Basingstoke: Macmillan, 1998, ch. 2.

21 Mechanic, D., 'Dilemmas in rationing healthcare services: the case for implicit rationing', *British Medical Journal,* Vol. 310, 1995, p. 1658.

22 Moran, 'Explaining change in the NHS: corporatism, closure and democratic capitalism', 1995, pp. 21-24.

23 Day, P. and Klein, R., 'Constitutional and distributional conflict in British medical politics: the case of general practice', 1911-91', *Political Studies*, Vol. 40, 1992, p. 468.

24 Klein, *The Politics of the NHS*, 1989, p. 82.

25 Dunleavy, P., 'Professional and policy change: notes towards a model of ideological corporatism', *Public Administration Bulletin*, Vol. 36, 1981, pp. 3-16; Dunleavy, P. and O'Leary, B., *Theories of the State: The Politics of Liberal Democracy,* London: Macmillan, 1987.

26 Merrison Committee, *Report of the Committee of Inquiry into the Regulation of the Medical Profession,*1975.

27 E.g. Elwell, H., *NHS: The Road to Recovery,* London: Centre for Policy Studies, 1988; Green, D.G., *Challenge to the NHS*, Hobart Paperback No. 23, London: Institute of Economic Affairs, 1986; Green, D.G., *Everyone a Private Patient,* Hobart Paperback No. 27, London: Institute of Economic Affairs, 1988; Letwin, O. and Redwood, J., *Britain's Biggest Enterprise: Ideas for Reform of the NHS,* London: Centre for Policy Studies, 1988.

28 Klein, R., 'From status to contract: the transformation of the British medical profession', in L' Etang, H. (ed.), *Health Care Provision Under Financial Constraint: a Decade of Change,* London: Royal Society of Medicine, 1990, p. 129.

29 Klein, R., 'The state and the profession: the politics of the double bed', *British Medical Journal,* Vol. 301, 1990, pp. 700-02.

30 Haywood, S. and Hunter, D.J., 'Consultative processes in health policy in the UK: a view from the centre', *Public Administration*, Vol. 69, 1982, pp. 143-62.

31 Lee-Potter, J., *A Damned Bad Business: the NHS Deformed,* London: Victor Gollancz, 1997.

32 Department of Health, *Working for Patients,* Cm. 555, London: HMSO, 1989, p. 40.

33 Hunter, D.J., 'From tribalism to corporatism: the managerial challenge to medical dominance', in Gabe, J., Kelleher, D. and Williams, G. (eds.), *Challenging Medicine*, London: Routledge, 1994; Klein, R., 'Big bang health care reform - does it work? The case of Britain's 1991 National Health Service reforms', *The Millbank Quarterly,* Vol. 73, No. 3, 1995, pp. 301-37.

34 Stacey, *Regulating British Medicine*, 1992, pp. 182-83.

35 Chief Medical Officer's Review Group, *Maintaining Medical Excellence: Review of Guidance on Doctors' Performance,* London: Department of Health, 1995, p. 7.

36 *The New NHS: Modern, Dependable,* Cm. 3807, London: The Stationery Office, 1997, p. 59.

37 Department of Health, 'NHS to have legal duty of ensuring quality for first time', press release 98/141, London: Department of Health, 13 April, 1998.

38 Department of Health, *A First Class Service: Quality in the New NHS*, London: Department of Health, 1998.

39 Department of Health, *A First Class Service*, 1998, para 3.44.

40 Department of Health, *A First Class Service*, 1998, para 2.27.

41 Merrison Committee, *Report of the Committee of Inquiry into the Regulation of the Medical Profession,* 1975, p. 5.

42 Evans, I., 'Conduct unbecoming–the MRC's approach', *British Medical Journal,* Vol. 316, 1998, pp. 1728-29.

43 Smith, R. 'The need for a national body for research misconduct', *British Medical Journal*, Vol. 316, 1998, pp. 1086-87.

44 Treasure, T., 'Lessons from the Bristol case', *British Medical Journal*, Vol. 316, 1998, pp. 1685-86.

45 Department of Health, *A First Class Service,* 1998, para 2.8.

46 Stacey, *Regulating British Medicine*, 1992, ch. 9.

47 Stacey, 'The GMC and professional accountability', 1989, p. 18.

48 Working Group on Specialist Medical Training, *Hospital Doctors: Training for the Future,* London: Department of Health (Calman Report), 1993.

49 General Medical Council, *The Recommendations on the Training of Specialists*, London: GMC, 1987.

50 Stacey, *Regulating British Medicine*, 1992, p. 121.

51 Stacey, *Regulating British Medicine*, 1992, pp. 250-51.

52 General Medical Council, *Professional Conduct and Discipline: Fitness to Practice,* London: GMC, 1993.

53 General Medical Council, *When Your Performance is Questioned*, London: GMC, 1997; General Medical Council, *The Management of Doctors with Problems: Referral to the GMC's Fitness to Practice Procedures,* London: GMC, 1997. See also Stacey, M., 'For public or profession? The new GMC performance procedures', *British Medical Journal*, Vol. 305, 1992, pp. 1085-87.

54 Keogh, B.E., Dussek, J., Watson, D., Magee, P. and Wheatley, D., 'Public confidence and cardiac surgical outcome', *British Medical Journal*, Vol. 316, 1998, p. 1760.

55 Keogh *et al*, 'Public confidence and cardiac surgical outcome', 1998.

56 Keogh *et al*, 'Public confidence and cardiac surgical outcome', 1998.

57 Department of Health, *A First Class Service*, 1998, ch. 2.

58 See e.g. Royal College of Physicians of London, *Medical Audit: A First Report, What, Why and How?,* London: Royal College of Physicians, 1989; Royal College of Surgeons of England, *Guidelines to Clinical Audit in Surgical Practice,* London: Royal College of Surgeons of England, 1989.

59 Keogh *et al,* 'Public confidence and cardiac surgical outcome', 1998, p. 1759.

60 British Medical Association, Academy of Medical Royal Colleges, Joint Consultants Committee, *Making Self-Regulation Work At The Local Level,* London: BMA, 1998, p. 4.

61 Barnes, R. and Hansted, K., 'Check up time', *Health Service Journal,* 21 May1998, pp. 26-27; Berger, A., 'Action on clinical audit: progress report', *British Medical Journal,* Vol. 316, 1998, pp. 1893-94; National Audit Office, *Clinical Audit in England,* HC 27, Session 1995-6, London: The Stationery Office, 1995.

62 Johnson, J.N., 'Making self-regulation credible', *British Medical Journal,* Vol. 316, 1998, p. 1848.

63 Johnson, 'Making self-regulation credible', 1998.

64 Warden, J., 'NHS hospital doctors face compulsory audit', *British Medical Journal,* Vol. 316, 1998, p. 1851.

65 Department of Health, *A First Class Service,* 1998: para 2.20.

66 Department of Health, *A First Class Service,* 1998: para 2.25.

67 GMC, *When Your Performance is Questioned,* 1997; GMC, *The Management of Doctors with Problems,* 1997.

68 Calman, K., *Continuing Medical Education,* consultation paper, London: Department of Health, p. 6.

69 Ward, S., 'Education for life', *British Medical Association, News Review,* 18-19 September 1994.

70 Calman, *Continuing Medical Education,* 1994, p. 11.

71 Department of Health, *A First Class Service,* 1998, para 3.12.

72 Department of Health, *A First Class Service,* 1998, para 3.14.

73 Allsop and Mulcahy, *Regulating Medical Work,* 1996, chs 2 and 3.

74 Donaldson, L.J., 'Doctors with problems in the NHS workforce', *British Medical Journal,* Vol. 309, 1994, pp. 1277-82.

75 CMO's Review Group, *Maintaining Medical Excellence,* 1995, p. 17.

76 British Medical Association, *CCSC Guidance for Senior Hospital Doctors on How to Deal with Concerns about the Performance of Colleagues,* London: BMA, 1997; British Medical Association, *CCSC Guidance for Developing the Role of Medical Directors,* London: BMA, 1997.

77 Johnson, 'Making self-regulation credible', 1998, p. 1848.

78 Department of Health, *A First Class Service*, 1998, para 2.26.

79 Stevens, R., *Medical Practice in Modern England: The Impact of Specialisation and State Medicine*, New Haven: Yale University Press, 1966, p. 284.

80 CMO's Review Group, *Maintaining Medical Excellence*, 1995, p. 3.

81 British Medical Association, Academy of Medical Royal Colleges, Joint Consultants Committee, *Making Self-Regulation Work At The Local Level*, London: BMA, 1998.

82 Horton, R., 'UK medicine: what are we to do?', *The Lancet*, Vol. 352, 1998, p. 1166.

83 Mayor, S., 'UK surgeons may undergo performance review every five years', *British Medical Journal*, Vol. 317, 1998, p. 1173.

84 Beecham, L. 'Consultants are wary of revalidation proposal', *British Medical Journal*, Vol. 317, 1998, p. 1087.

85 Salter, B., 'Medicine and the state: redefining the concordat', *Public Policy and Administration*, Vol. 10, No. 3, 1995, pp. 60-87.

Meg Stacey

1 Larkin, G., 'State control and the Health Professions', in Johnson, T., Larkin, G. and Saks, M., *Health Professions and the State in Europe*, Routledge: London and New York, 1995.

2 Smith, R., 'All changed, changed utterly', *British Medical Journal*, Vol. 316, 1998, p. 1917.

3 Stacey, M., *Regulating British Medicine: The General Medical Council*, Chichester: Wiley, 1992.

4 Cooper, D., Lowe, A., Puxty, A., Robson, K. and Willmott, H., 'Regulating the UK accountancy profession: episodes in the relation between the profession and the state', paper presented at the Economic and Social Research Council Conference on Corporatism at the Policy Studies Institute, January 1988, cited in Macdonald, K., *The Sociology of the Professions*, London: Sage, 1995, p. 10.

5 Larson, M., *The Rise of Professionalism: A Sociological Analysis*, London: University of California Press, 1977.

6 Moran, M. and Wood, B., *States, Regulation and the Medical Profession*, Buckingham: Open University Press, 1993, pp. 17-19; Allsop, J. and Mulcahy, L., *Regulating Medical Work: Formal and Informal*, Buckingham: Open University Press, 1996, pp. 8-9.

7 Macdonald, *The Sociology of the Professions*, 1995, p. 58.

8 Jarausch, K.H., 'The German professions in history and theory', in Cocks, G. and Jarausch, K.H. (eds.), *German Professions 1850-1950*, New York and Oxford: Oxford University Press, 1990, pp. 9-24.

9   Moran and Wood, *States, Regulation and the Medical Profession*, 1993, pp. 17-19.

10 Allsop and Mulcahy, *Regulating Medical Work*, 1996, pp. 8-9.

11 Moran and Wood, *States, Regulation and the Medical Profession*, 1993.

12 Irvine, D.H., 'Dysfunctional doctors; the General Medical Council's new approach', in Rosenthal, M.M., Mulcahy, L. and Lloyd-Bostock, S., *Medical Mishaps: Pieces of the Puzzle*, Buckingham: Open University Press, 1999, p. 186.

13 Stacey, *Regulating British Medicine,* 1992, ch. 13; Robinson, J., 'A patients voice at the GMC: a lay member's view of the GMC', *Health Rights*, Report No. 1, London: Health Rights, 1988.

14 See her account in Robinson, J., 'The price of deceit: the reflections of an advocate', in Rosenthal *et al*, *Medical Mishaps*, 1999, pp. 250-51.

15 General Medical Council, *Good Medical Practice*, London: General Medical Council, 1998.

16 General Medical Council, *Good Medical Practice*, 1998, p. 9.

17 Stacey, *Regulating British Medicine*, 1992.

18 Irvine, D.H., 'The performance of doctors I: professionalism and self-regulation in a changing world', *British Medical Journal*, Vol. 314, 1997, pp. 1540-42; Irvine, D., 'The performance of doctors II: maintaining good practice, protecting patients for poor performance', *British Medical Journal*, Vol. 314, 1997, pp. 1613-15; Irvine, 'Dysfunctional doctors; the General Medical Council's new approach', 1999.

19 General Medical Council, *Good Medical Practice,* London: GMC 1995.

20 Delamothe, T., 'Who killed Cock Robin?', *British Medical Journal*, Vol. 316, 1998, p. 1757.

21 The President spelled out the following broad implications of the inquiry:
    1   The need for clearly understood clinical standards
    2   How clinical competence and technical expertise are assessed and evaluated
    3   Who carries the responsibility in team-based care
    4   The training of doctors in advanced procedures
    5   How to approach the so-called learning curve of doctors undertaking established procedures
    6   The reliability and validity of the data used to monitor doctors' personal performance
    7   The use of medical audit
    8   The appreciation of the importance of factors, other than purely clinical ones, that can affect clinical judgement, performance and outcome

9   The responsibility of a consultant to take appropriate action in response to concerns about his or her performance

10 The factors which seem to discourage openness and frankness about doctors' personal performance

22 Department of Health, *The New NHS: Modern, Dependable*, London: Department of Health,1997; Department of Health, *A First Class Service: Quality in the New NHS*, London: Department of Health, 1998.

23 See Salter, B., 'Who Rules? The New Politics of Medical Regulation', forthcoming, *Social Science and Medicine*.

24 Treasure, T., 'Lessons from the Bristol case', *British Medical Journal*, Vol. 316, 1998, pp. 1685-86.

25 Kennedy, I., *The Unmasking of Medicine*, London: Granada, 1983; Rosenthal, M.M., *Dealing with Medicine Malpractice*, London: Tavistock, 1987, Rosenthal, M.M., *The Incompetent Doctor: Behind Closed Doors*, Buckingham: Open University Press, 1995; Smith, R., 'The day of judgement comes closer', *British Medical Journal*, 1989, Vol. 298, pp. 1241-44; Stacey, M., 'The GMC and professional accountability', *Public Policy and Administration*, 1989, Vol. 4, No. 1, pp. 12-27; Stacey, *Regulating British Medicine*, 1992; Allsop, J. and Mulcahy, L., *Regulating Medical Work: Formal and Informal Controls*, Buckingham: Open University Press, 1996.

26 Brandt, T., 'Sociological approaches to the professions', *Acta Socioligca*, 1988, 31:2.

27 Johnson, J.N., 'Making self-regulation credible', *British Medical Journal*, 1998; Vol. 316, pp. 1847-8.

28 Stacey, M., 'The case for and against medical self-regulation', Paper to the Second International Conference on Medical Regulation, Melbourne, Australia, Mimeo, 1996, p. 23.

29 Klein, R., 'Competence, professional self regulation, and the public interest, *British Medical Journal*, 1998, Vol. 316, pp. 1742.

William Pickering

1   Pickering, W.G., 'Kindness, prescribed and natural, in medicine', *Journal of Medical Ethics*, 1997, Vol. 23, pp. 116-18.

2   Moyez, J., 'Autonomy: the need for limits', *Journal of Medical Ethics*, 1996,Vol. 22, pp. 340-43.

3   Moyez, 'Autonomy: the need for limits', 1996.

4   Pickering, W.G., 'How to control misuse of the health services', *British Medical Journal*, November 1996, Vol. 313, pp. 1408-09.

5   Pickering, W.G., 'Does medical treatment mean patient benefit?', *Lancet*, 1996, Vol. 347, pp. 379-80.

6 Department of Health, *A First Class Service: Quality in the New NHS*, London: Department of Health, June 1998.

7 *Performance Procedures. A Summary of Current Proposals*, London: GMC, 178 Portland Street, London W1N 6JE (tel: 020 7580 7642), 1997.

8 'Health Service Commissioner for England, Scotland and Wales', *Annual Report 1995-96*, London: HMSO, 1997.

9 Dental Practice Board, Compton Place Road, Eastbourne, E. Sussex BN20 8AD (tel: 01323 417000).

10 Martin, I. *et al.*, 'Delays in the diagnosis of oesophageal cancer: a consecutive case series', *British Medical Journal*, February 1997, Vol. 314, p. 467.

11 Lakshmanan, Hershey, and Breslau, 'Hospital admissions caused by iatrogenic disease', *Archives of Internal Medicine*, October 1986, Vol. 146, pp. 1931-34.

12 The Committee on Safety of Medicines Yellow Card Scheme.

13 Rawlins, M.D. 'Pharmacovigilance: paradise lost, regained or postponed?', *Journal of the Royal College of Physicians of London*, January/February 1995, Vol. 29 No. 1.

14 Langman, M., 'Peptic ulcer complications and the use of non-aspirin non-steroidal anti-inflammatory drugs', *Adverse Drug Reaction Bulletin*, 1986, Vol. 120, pp. 448-51.

15 Pickering W.G., 'The negligent treatment of the medical anecdote', *British Medical Journal*, 6 June 1992, Vol. 304, p. 1516.

16 Steel, K., 'Iatrogenic disease in a medical service', *Journal of American Geriatric Society*, 1984, Vol. 32, pp. 445-49.

17 Pickering, 'Does medical treatment mean patient benefit?', 1996.

18 Rawlins, 'Pharmacovigilance: paradise lost, regained or postponed?', 1995.

19 Pickering, W.G., 'Patient satisfaction: an imperfect measurement of quality medicine', *Journal of Medical Ethics*, 1993, Vol. 19, pp. 121-22.

20 *Being Heard*, London: Department of Health, 1994, paras. 52-56; Vincent, C. *et al.*, 'Why do people sue doctors? A study of patients and relatives taking legal action', *Lancet*, Vol. 343, 25 June 1994, pp. 1609-13.

21 Department of Health, *A First Class Service*, June 1998.

Index

Independence

The Institute for the Study of Civil Society is a registered educational charity (No. 1036909). The ISCS is financed from a variety of private sources to avoid over-reliance on any single or small group of donors.

All publications are independently refereed and referees' comments are passed on anonymously to authors. All the Institute's publications seek to further its objective of promoting the advancement of learning. The views expressed are those of the authors, not of the ISCS.